REAL-WORLD FITNESS

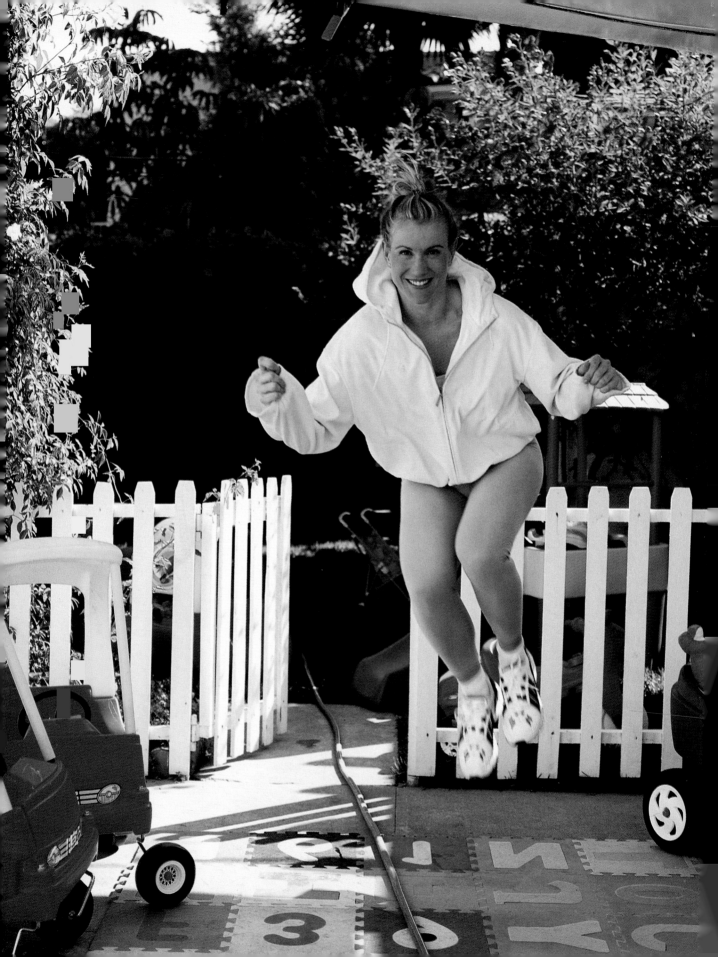

REAL-WORLD FITNESS

KATHY KAEHLER *with*

DR. CHERYL K. OLSON

Golden Books
New York

To my clients who contributed to this book: Thank you for your time and thoughts. I know each of your experiences, your contributions, will click with someone else and move them closer to a healthier, more active life.

Special thanks to my assistant, Kathleen Ingle, for keeping all the loose ends together.
—K.K.

Thanks to my very patient husband and son.
—C.K.O.

This book is not intended to be a substitute for professional medical advice. The reader should regularly consult a physician regarding any matter concerning his or her health and before beginning this or any other exercise program.

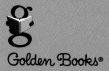

Golden Books®
888 Seventh Avenue
New York, NY 10106

Copyright © 1999 by Kathy Kaehler
All rights reserved, including the right of reproduction
in whole or in part in any form.

Golden Books® and colophon are trademarks
of Golden Books Publishing Co., Inc.

Designed by Red Herring Design
Photographs by Mike Russ Photography
Manufactured in the United States of America

10 9 8 7 6 5 4 3 2 1

The Library of Congress Cataloging-in-Publication Data

Kaehler, Kathy.
    Real-world fitness / Kathy Kaehler with Cheryl K. Olson.
       p. cm.
    Incudes bibliographical references (p.).
    ISBN 1-58238-026-0
    1. Physical Fitness. 2. Exercise. I. Olson, Cheryl K.
II. Title.
GV1.K34 1999
613.7--dc21

                                    98-37293
                                    CIP

CONTENTS

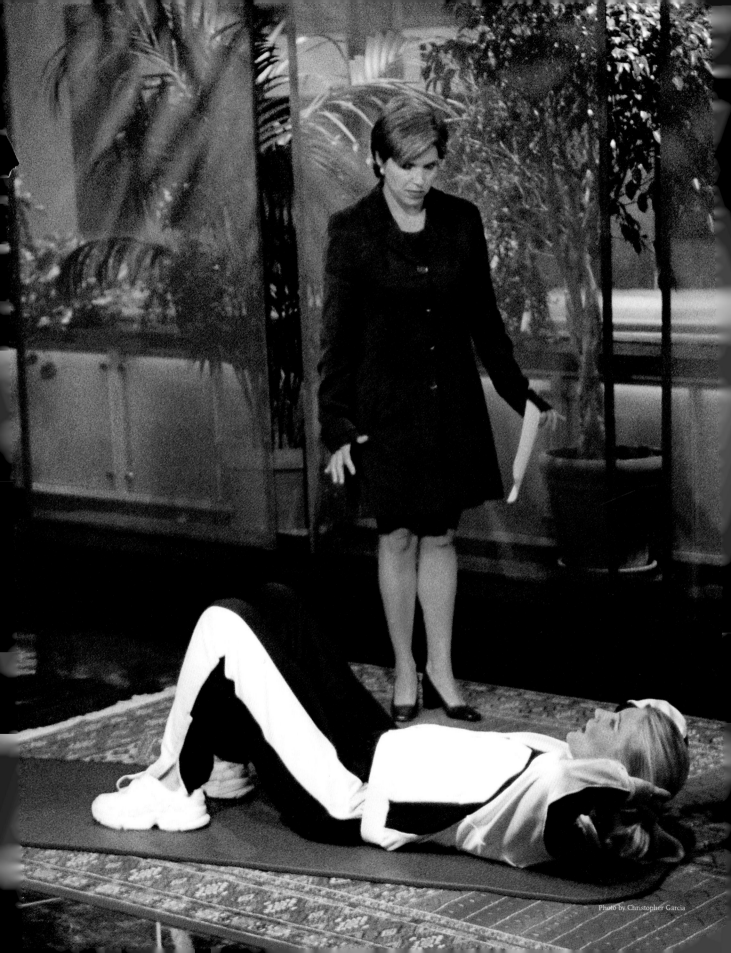

Photo by Christopher Garcia

INTRODUCTION
BEHIND THE SCENES AND BEFORE THE CAMERA

MOST FITNESS BOOKS ASSUME THAT WORKING OUT SHOULD BE THE TOP PRIORITY IN YOUR LIFE—AND THAT YOU MUST DO IT "RIGHT." YOU STRUGGLE TO FIND TIME TO DRIVE TO A GYM FOR A 45-MINUTE CLASS, SHOWER, AND DRIVE BACK. YOU PUZZLE OVER DIFFICULT ROUTINES. YOUR MUSCLES HURT AND THE DOUGHNUTS CALL YOUR NAME. PRETTY SOON, YOUR GOOD INTENTIONS RUN OUT OF GAS AND YOU'VE GIVEN UP ON EXERCISE AGAIN.

Coaching, teaching, and putting together individualized programs for my clients over the years have taught me a lot about human nature and about working with people who don't naturally have exercise in their lives.

I understand the struggle of someone who doesn't exercise but wants to—the battles with determination and focus. I know how to get her to the point where exercise becomes as natural as brushing her teeth, as it is for me.

> What I find most fascinating about Kathy is that every time she comes on *Today*, she has a way of breaking up what could be tedious and even complicated into a very digestible segment.
>
> It's never something where you've gotta go out and buy some incredible piece of equipment to help you accomplish this. Instead, it's using something like elastic and a book.
>
> She's just amazing at coming up with simple ways to get you A) thinking about fitness and B) accomplishing something that seems minor but fetches major results if you stick to it.
>
> —*Matt Lauer*

A lot of people can teach you to do perfect leg lifts. I've learned that communication, and understanding how you get someone to do it and *keep doing it*, are just as important.

I also know from personal experience how tough it can be to fit exercise into a hectic schedule. I train people all day, but it's hard to find time to work out at my own pace and do what I need for me.

Every other Thursday, I train my morning clients, pack, and then leave Los Angeles on a 4:00 P.M.-to-midnight flight to New York. I grab a few hours of sleep, and then it's "Oh, my God, is that the alarm?" The car from *Today* picks me up at six.

I'm usually *really* tired. But being on TV gets my adrenaline going. From day one when I walked into the *Today* studio, it felt like one big happy family. Everyone is warm and friendly and easy to talk to. And after doing this for years, even every other week, I still get excited to see people. I love visiting with Katie Couric, Matt Lauer, Al Roker, Ann Curry, and the rest. It's also fun to meet the celebrities out promoting their new films.

Each time I try to make my segment better than the last. How can I bring my energy and motivation to the viewer? How can Katie and I build our rapport and make the segment useful and informative—and maybe a little silly? (It's hard not to get silly with Katie.)

I've done segments on a variety of topics for *Today*. I did one on exercises you can do in bed, like a chest pullover. (Stick a five- or ten-pound weight on the floor, just under the foot of your bed. Lie on your back on the bed—with your head at its foot—grab the weight, and pull it up and over you, down toward your belly button—then back again behind you. Restful, isn't it?)

I've made Katie do all kinds of things. We did one segment just before Christmas in which I showed her how to save time by doing stretches while wrapping gifts. (Get on the floor, with legs apart in a straddle position; put the wrap and tape in front of you. Between each present, bend over and do some stretching. It gets rid of that holiday-time tension in your upper and lower body.) So there we were on the floor, wrapping presents with our legs splayed out!

The *Today* producers always tell me, "Just do something that doesn't require equipment. Things you can do around the home, with a stroller, stairs, a wall ... " And one day I thought, It would be great to have all of these ideas in a book. I

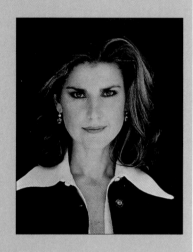

A friend of mine said, "You need to talk to Kathy Kaehler." Kathy just came so highly recommended. I think we'd been working out for 30 minutes when I said, "Are you on *Today*?" I didn't know she was the woman on *Today* whom I admired so much.

—*Peri Gilpin*

envisioned a book that the busy people who watch me on *Today* or read my column in *Women's Sports and Fitness* could flip through on their own schedule, picking out things they could easily do, whatever their daily routines.

A Day in My Life

Fortunately I'm a morning person, because I leave the house between five and six o'clock. I throw on a T-shirt, bike shorts, and tennis shoes and grab some oatmeal or a protein shake. I'll sneak a peek at my sleeping toddlers, Cooper and Payton. If I don't wake them up, it makes the morning easier for them, and I know I'll get to be with them later.

The first person I see is usually Michelle Pfeiffer. Through many personal changes (single woman to wife to mother of two) and all her movie roles, Michelle has stayed committed to her workouts with me. For an hour, we go running or in-line skating on the boardwalk at the beach, do circuit training in her gym, hike, do step aerobics—my goal is to keep things interesting and varied for her, since we've trained together for so long.

"There are always a million-and-one reasons why you can't exercise today," says Michelle. "For me, even if it means losing sleep, I really have to get it done before I do anything, otherwise I'll find one of those reasons not to do it."

By 7:15, I'm at Julianne Phillips's house, doing step aerobics. "I'm very competitive with myself," admits Julianne, "and to work with somebody like Kathy, who's equally strong or better—that keeps me motivated. I like to break a sweat, and work all those parts that I want to keep lifted—the ones that must defy gravity."

Then I'm back in the car (you spend a lot of time in cars in Los Angeles), driving to the next person. Often I head to a private Hollywood gym called Muscle Under, where I train clients like Nancy Travis, Alfre Woodard, Samuel L. Jackson, Jennifer Aniston, and Peri Gilpin until 1:00.

"Kathy understands what I'm going for and keeps me on track," Peri says. "She's always teaching me little things I can do at home, even while I'm reading scripts or talking on the phone. She thinks about what someone's life is like and takes it from there, not 'You must take an hour-and-a-half out of your day and go do this.'"

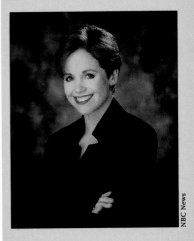

NBC News

Kathy is a real person, and I think people appreciate that and relate to her. She emphasizes good health, strong bodies—not waifdom—and I think that is the most compelling reason to get in shape.

—*Katie Couric*

I try to grab 30 minutes to eat lunch. Sometimes I'll have a luxury day, with two hours off. If there's time, I'll zip home to see my twins. Occasionally one or two clients will cancel, and I can meet my kids at the park. (That's the nice part of being my own boss.)

I see more clients, such as Lisa Kudrow or Rita Wilson, in the afternoon. Not all of my clients have names you'd recognize: they include attorneys, housewives, and a hotel owner. But they're all good people and (most days) fun to work with. And they all have the same basic needs.

People often ask me, "What's it like training all those TV and movie stars?" They're the same as anyone else. All my clients want to get stronger, tone up their bodies, look better, be fitter for what they want and need to do in their lives. All that's different about my famous clients is the work they do.

To balance all this work, I squeeze in time to take care of me. Once a week, I'll take an acting class, which is like a kind of playful therapy for me. I also try to fit in a class, such as Tae Bo or boxing, and get a weekly facial.

My last client's done at 6:30 every day, so I have time with my family in the evenings. With the kids' schedule the way it is, we try to have dinner at 7:00 when I get home. I spend nearly all my time with my boys from when I come home Friday until Monday morning. (Sometimes I even get to talk with my husband!) Then I try to get to bed early, at least by 10:30.

Before I had the kids, I'd go once a week to a celebrity party or a movie opening. (That's how I met my husband: attending the premiere of *Other People's Money* with Penelope Ann Miller.) Now we go out only once or twice a month. It has to be important to miss time with the twins.

Most nights I'm home, giving my kids baths, doing laundry for four . . . you get the picture. Sometimes I can grab just 10 minutes at night to jump on my bike, run on the treadmill, or do some sit-ups. But, as this book will demonstrate, grabbing exercise when and where you can really does count.

"There are always a million-and-one reasons why you can't exercise today," says Michelle Pfeiffer. *"For me, even if it means losing sleep, I really have to get it done before I do anything, otherwise I'll find one of those reasons not to do it."*

Why I Do What I Do

I've been involved in athletics and fitness for the majority of my life. My mom says I was always the fastest kid on the playground, challenging the boys because I could already beat all the girls. In college, I was a dance/physical education major, going out for volleyball, basketball, and track.

When I graduated, I was lucky enough to snag an internship at Coors in Colorado, home of one of the nation's first corporate fitness programs. That gave me my first taste of one-on-one fitness training.

I worked with people who didn't have much activity or exercise in their lives, creating programs that took into account their desires and constraints. Through my coaching and teaching, I'd see them blossom. I found that I was good at helping people build that determination to change. I learned how to get my clients to that point where exercise felt as natural and regular as getting dressed in the morning.

When I completed my internship, I found work in Denver's booming health club industry. That's where I met my friend and mentor Dr. Daniel Kosich, working with him in a club designing one-on-one training programs. He later left the club to take a job with Jane Fonda's organization.

Six months after he'd left, he called me and said, "There's a job that's opened up at Jane's spa. I told her about you, and she'd like to meet you." Wow!

Soon after, I flew from Denver to Los Angeles, where Daniel picked me up and drove me to Santa Barbara. I hadn't been to California since I was seven years old. We drove way up in the mountains, along this curvy road, and pulled up before a huge gate with a big sign: Laurel Springs. Laurel Springs was like a country farm estate, with barns for animals and lodge-style buildings. We pulled up to this little house, got out of the car, and I saw Jane coming across the lawn. I remember this feeling of sweaty palms and erratic breathing: she was the first famous person I'd ever met.

I think Jane took all the star-struckness I'd ever have in my life away that day. I haven't felt that way since, even when I've met Barbra Streisand, Cher, Arnold Schwarzenegger, and other big names in the course of my training work.

> If you meet Kathy, don't ever try to take her in a fight. She's the strongest woman I've ever known. She could probably beat up about three-quarters of my male friends.
>
> Not that she'd ever do that.
>
> —Al Roker

My interview with Jane started with a hike, and she basically kicked my butt. I remember climbing this hill, thinking that for sure I could outdo her—she was fifty and I was a fit woman in my late twenties, after all—and there she was, way ahead of me. I tried not to let her see how hard I was breathing.

Next, she had me teach her a private aerobics class. That took all the nerve and brains I could muster, to teach the queen of aerobics a one-on-one class. At this point I was exhausted, but Jane went on to the pool and swam some laps.

We finished up in the gym, discussing my history with fitness. Since Laurel Springs was designed as a spa for people in the entertainment industry, Jane explained that many clients would be veterans of crazy diets, exercise fads, and other obsessions related to food and working out. She was looking for someone who could bring some honesty and realism to teaching clients how to change their lives through healthy eating and exercise.

Jane also talked about her personal experiences, and it turned out that we'd had some similar problems along the way (yes, I went through a phase of starving myself and taking diet pills in college—before I learned it didn't work). We hit it off.

The next day, she called and said I had the job. That's what brought me into this celebrity realm and changed my life. In the year I spent at Laurel Springs, I worked one-on-one with a number of Jane's friends, including Rue McClanahan, Sharon Gless, Melanie Griffith, and Ally Sheedy.

When the Laurel Springs spa closed, I "jumped off the diving board" and nervously started calling up the people I had trained. It so happened that Melanie Griffith needed someone to help her prepare for *Working Girl*. And that's how I got started as an independent celebrity fitness trainer.

I never could have planned all the opportunies I've had. (Not to mention finding my wonderful husband, Billy, and having our twins.) Who could have anticipated things this good? It was partly the right place at the right time, but I think it's also that internal flame, that motivation to do better, which is what prompted me to write to Katie Couric and get hired by NBC's *Today*. In my case, that energy comes from being physical and helping others become more physical.

A Little Fitness Counts a Lot

Especially around New Year's resolution time, people will come to me and say, "I can't live the way I've been living anymore. I need to start over. I'll exercise every day. I'm going to change the way I eat"—they want to change everything. This fervor may last a week, maybe a month, but the point is, it doesn't last. They'll go back to their old habits. Nobody can be "perfect" forever.

There are people who can exercise 45 to 60 minutes, 5 days a week, and that's fantastic. They won't have as many problems with life's ups and downs. (If you're in this category, you'll find ideas for varying your routine and staying motivated in this book.)

But many more people feel they can spare only 20 or even 10 minutes here and there. And they've heard that if you can't run and sweat for at least half an hour most days, exercise is a waste of time. So they throw up their hands and say, "I just won't exercise at all." Big mistake.

"That prescription of structured, intensive exercise is still good," says Andrea Dunn, Ph.D., associate director of epidemiology and clinical applications at the Cooper Institute for Aerobics Research in Dallas. "But the thing is, most people aren't doing it. And I assume they won't do it, because if they would, more of us would be regularly physically active. And that's just not the case."

"With exercise, something is much better than nothing," says Kenneth Cooper, M.D. Need proof? For years, Dr. Cooper and his colleagues at the Cooper Institute have been studying the effects of physical fitness (or lack of it) on health and longevity. In 1989, the *Journal of the American Medical Association* published the results of the Institute's groundbreaking study of over 13,000 men and women.

"We found that if you looked at the least-fit 20 percent versus the top 20 percent, the decrease in death rates from all causes was 65 percent," says Dr. Cooper. "But by moving from the bottom 20 percent to the next-highest 20 percent, you got most of that benefit." In other words, even a moderate amount of exercise drastically reduces your odds of illness and early death.

1996 SURGEON GENERAL'S REPORT ON PHYSICAL ACTIVITY AND HEALTH

Only 15 percent of Americans hit the gym or the trail for 20 minutes–plus of intensive aerobic activity on three or more days of the week. The majority of people, 60 percent, aren't regularly active. They get out for the occasional brisk walk, maybe a weekend game of tennis or pickup basketball. The final 25 percent? They exercise by walking from the car to the house.

People don't realize that you can accomplish a lot with 10 minutes here and there, if you keep at it. Says Dr. Cooper, "Ten minutes of walking in the morning and 10 in the afternoon plus walking up and down the stairs and back and forth to the car will probably move you from the bottom 20 percent to that next level."

As I'll show you in this book, grabbing exercise when and where you can really does count. Whether your goal is to climb stairs without panting, drop a dress size, feel more attractive and confident, or reduce symptoms of stress, I can help you make it happen.

I'll give you dozens of ways to create a personal squeeze-it-in fitness plan that will truly produce results and be easy to maintain. Fitness is about alternatives. It should fit into your lifestyle; you don't have to build your life around the gym.

There are no rigid rules here. You can reward yourself with a brownie at the end of the day if you've done something physical to balance it. There's no need to deprive yourself of anything.

Exercise can help you balance your life, not steal time from it. Getting your spouse or kids involved in your fitness routine, as some of my clients do, creates extra fun time together. I'll show you ideas and ways to get active that can be safely started by people of any age or fitness level.

This book will help you take the focus off how you "should" exercise and how you "should" look, and put it on the more meaningful benefits of exercise. How does fitness change you emotionally? Playing basketball with your child is a good way to burn calories, sure, but it also makes you both happy. Exercise is not about having a perfect figure (an impossible and highly subjective goal anyway). It's about having a body that feels good.

> What impressed me about Kathy is that she had an athletic, healthy-looking body. You know how some people train for the sake of training? They walk around looking carved, but those aren't useful bodies for living in today's world. What impresses me is a fit and strong body that looks practical, like it's going to help you do things.
>
> —Alfre Woodard

A WINNING ATTITUDE

Not long ago, researchers at Oxford University's Department of Public Health
gave about 2000 people a health checkup. Participants were asked,
"Would you like to get more exercise?" Those who said yes were asked about
what made it hard for them to do that. Some people named "internal barriers":
I'm too busy. I'm no good at sports. I'm too lazy. I don't enjoy exercise.

Others mentioned "external barriers": My friends or partner are not
interested in exercise. There isn't a sports facility close by. I can't afford
to go, or I have no way to get there, or I have no child care.
Finally, some people chose both internal and external barriers.

When the subjects were re-interviewed three years later, the researchers
found something surprising. The people who hadn't gotten moving were not
the ones who couldn't afford the gym, or faced any of the other external barriers.
(Maybe recognizing those barriers helped them find solutions.)
No, the ones who were still sitting and wishing they could change
came mostly from the group whose only barriers were in their heads!

So don't let a hopeless attitude get in the way
of the fit and happy person you want to be.

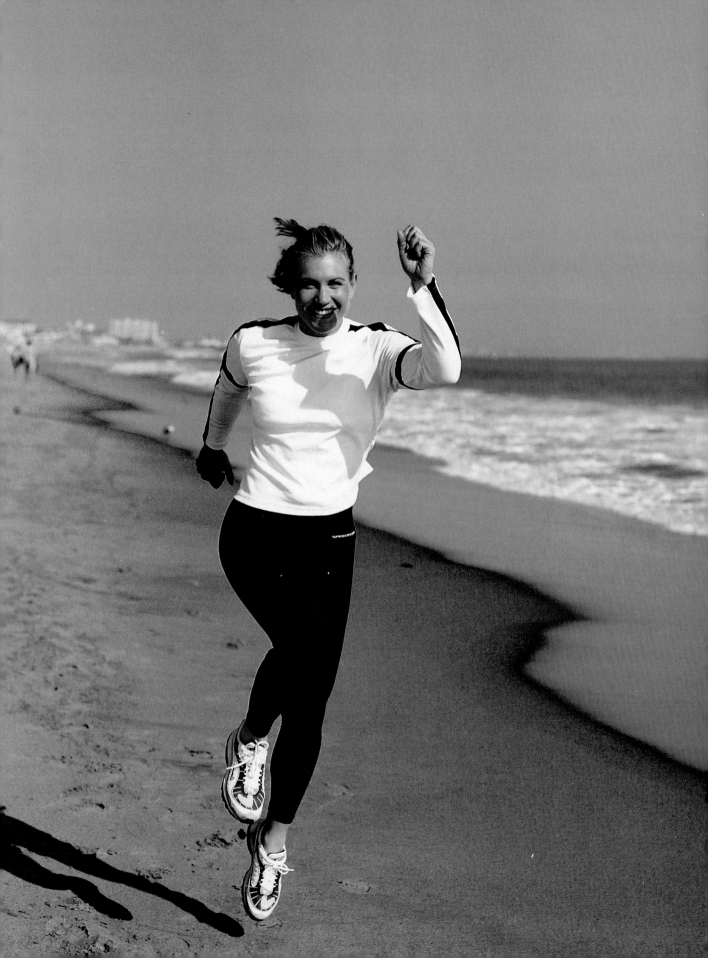

1 GETTING STARTED

Most summers, I go to my family's cabin in Ontario and get some uninterrupted time with my family, especially with my twins. One day I was watching my mom play with them. She was singing that old song, "This is the way we wash our clothes, wash our clothes..." and acting it out. It got me thinking.

Remember those old scrubbing boards and wringer washers? It took hours to do laundry that way. It was just a heartbeat ago in the history of humans that we were farming, wringing out clothes, carrying heavy loads, walking everywhere. People back then didn't think about exercise, because they were naturally so active. They had all this stuff to do.

Today, we sit and push buttons. We stare at our computers and televisions. There's that handy car waiting to take us places; no need to walk or bike. We have elevators and escalators to replace the stairs; we stand on belts that carry us through airports. Few of us beat eggs by hand, crank open the garage door, or push a no-motor lawn mower. At home, at work, and almost everywhere we go, circumstances and machines discourage our bodies from moving.

No wonder the latest government stats show we're getting fatter. More than *one in three adults over 19* now weigh too much! Adding regular physical activity to our lives is more difficult, and more vital, than ever before. I'm not saying I want to scrub dirty clothes by hand the way my great-grandmother did. But we need to find ways to get our bodies moving.

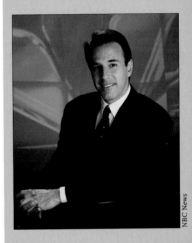

NBC News

When I started at NBC, the demands of the job were tremendous. I was working both ends of the clock: doing *Today* in the morning and anchoring the local news at night. So I was a mess. I was always either working, napping, or eating. And I kinda fell away from fitness.

—Matt Lauer

FITNESS SHOULD NOT HURT

When new clients call me—whether they want to lose weight, change their body, get ready for a role, or just get fit and stronger—they already have a preconceived idea of what that's going to take. Some think it's a lot more difficult than it really is. Exercise means sweat, exhaustion, and pain, right? While sweat is optional, the others definitely are out.

A lot of people still have the idea that you have to be red in the face and out of breath. Those are totally unnecessary, even counterproductive, in making exercise effective.

"I talk about 'activity' instead of 'exercise,'" says exercise physiologist Dr. Daniel Kosich, "because for most people, 'exercise' and 'fitness' are not real positive terms. They conjure up images of struggle and fatigue, and effort beyond comfort."

And activity is more than exercise. Formal exercise, such as a step aerobics class, does work off more calories in a short time. But don't underestimate the power of daily activity: getting your body moving whenever the chance presents itself. "Ten calories here, 15 there—it quickly adds up," says Dr. Kosich.

As an exercise psychologist, Andrea Dunn has helped hundreds of people add activity to their lives. "One of the major barriers to exercise that people describe is lack of time," says Dr. Dunn. "But it's actually a lack of time-management skills."

I think it actually goes beyond that, to a lack of clear and healthy priorities. I hear people bitch and moan about feeling fat, hating how they look in clothes, being tired and stressed, not having enough strength . . . but if you're not doing anything about it, you're obviously not making change a priority. If you were, you'd find some way during your 24 hours to exercise or be active. If it's not a priority, you won't be alert to those opportunities: Here's the elevator, but there are the stairs, and stairs are what I need.

"Too busy? Here I am, 67 years of age, working 60 to 70 hours every week," says Dr. Kenneth Cooper. "I'm on the road about 50 percent of the time. And I haven't missed more than three consecutive days doing something aerobic in the last 39 years. If I can work it out, you can."

"Most people want to be active but just don't think they can be," Dr. Dunn adds. "People get in these black-and-white thinking modes about being physically active: for example, thinking the only thing that really counts is going to a gym and being vigorously active, and that other approaches won't work for them."

There's no reason to segregate exercise mentally or physically from real life. It shouldn't be "go the gym, do a class, rush home, plop down—done moving for today." For example, Jennifer Aniston doesn't waste time traveling to a gym; she runs up and down the hills in her neighborhood. We made that into a great, fast aerobic workout. (When we came back, our legs were shaking!) The point is, you don't need a fancy gym or expensive equipment to get fit and healthy.

"With technology, we've been engineering activity out of our lives," reminds Dr. Andrea Dunn. "But if we can engineer it out, we can engineer it back in."

You can do that with a more formal exercise program (see Chapter 5, "Eight Weeks to a Show-Off Body"), or by sneaking in more movement throughout your daily schedule (see Chapter 2, "Stealth Fitness").

Why Do You Want to Get Fit?
Benefits of Exercise

There are many excellent reasons to get serious about fitness.

"I felt lethargic," Al Roker recalls. "I didn't feel like I had any strength, like I was deteriorating. And my wife and I were trying to have a baby; that was a factor. And not dropping dead from a heart attack.

"I get up at 4:30 A.M.," says Al. "I have the *Today* show from seven to nine, I have other responsibilities, and then I do the 5:00 news in New York. It's a long day, and I needed to do something to increase my stamina."

For Samuel L. Jackson, it was feeling the passage of time. "It's disconcerting to realize that you're getting older, and some of the things you thought you could do, you can't do," he says. "I used to do 100 push-ups. Then one day I thought, Now wait a minute, I can't do 20 push-ups fast. I wanted to feel stronger.

"Also, sometimes I think I'll do one of these action films, and I want to look halfway in shape," he adds, "in case I have to take my clothes off, or some of them come off."

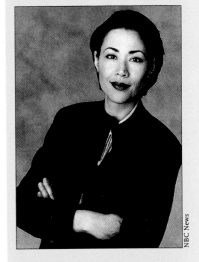

Ann Curry

Becoming a mother did it for Nancy Travis. "I'd had a baby, and everything was in a different place, all reconfigured," she says. "I wanted to lose the excess and build up some stamina."

Sometimes people are motivated by "use it or lose it." Ann Curry, who reports the news on *Today* (and occasionally does fitness segments with me), says, "A friend of mine needed to have a pin put in her knee. She could never run again. I realized it was a privilege just to move."

"One of the motivating reasons that I'm physically active is that I want to function better in old age," says Dr. Andrea Dunn of the Cooper Institute. "Physical activity is a key to maintaining independence."

Researchers at the University of Michigan's School of Public Health have found that shocking numbers of American women in their forties and fifties have the strength and fitness levels you'd expect to see in great-grandmothers. This doesn't mean they can't last through an aerobics class; they have trouble carrying groceries, climbing stairs, and walking around the block!

Fitness is not a moral issue (there's no shame in having higher priorities than exercise), but it is a *freedom issue*. When you sit around, put on weight, and lose muscle tone, you surrender choices and lose independence. A 1998 study from Stanford University showed that for both men and women, sitting around increases your risk of disability, at any age.

While we're talking research, consider a 1996 study by Cooper Institute researchers Steven Blair and James Kampert. They found that the two outstanding risks for early death among women were low fitness levels and smoking. Even women who were overweight, smoked, or had other health problems lived longer if they did regular, moderate exercise.

According to the Surgeon General's report, here are some of the health problems you can avoid or minimize if you're regularly physically active: heart disease, diabetes, high blood pressure, colon cancer, feelings of depression and anxiety, excess weight, weak bones and joints, and falls (which can cause deadly fractures among older women). Exercise may even protect against breast cancer (the jury's still out on that). When you add better-fitting clothes and that sexy feeling of confidence you get from being active, what are you waiting for?

Thin Is Not Fit

When you page through a magazine and see a beautiful, lean model, you probably think she's got no worries in the health and fitness department. You might be right, but you could be fooled. Looking great in photographs tells you little about a person's condition.

Claudia Schiffer is a good example. A few years ago, a friend told me that Claudia planned to make some exercise videos (as several supermodels were doing), and needed a fitness expert to do it with her. I'd heard there were four or five other trainers coming to be interviewed. But as it turned out, I didn't need to audition: Claudia had already decided on me based on my first step-aerobics video, *Kathy Kaehler's Fitness System.*

The point is, people would assume, "Well, she's thin— she doesn't have to do anything."

"What intrigued me about Kathy was her warm personality," Claudia recalls. "I felt like I knew her."

Claudia had personal as well as professional goals: "I wanted to tone my body, shape up my thin arms—and also lift my metabolism, because I love to eat." We talked about how she envisioned the video workouts, and how she wanted to look.

Every night for a month, I commuted to Las Vegas for our training sessions. I immediately realized that even though she was super-slim, her body urgently needed work. She was just not ready to do what she'd planned for her video. I normally have people pushing eight- to ten-pound weights 15 times for upper body workouts, and Claudia couldn't even do 8 reps with a three-pound weight. She lasted barely 10 minutes on the Stairmaster.

"Kathy worked me to death," says Claudia. "There were times I asked myself what I was doing, but I definitely needed it. I had no endurance, and I really needed more muscle and strength.

"I was a little afraid, because I thought it would be too hard or painful. But I wasn't embarrassed to sometimes let Kathy know I was getting tired."

In our first video, for arms, I included a segment on push-ups. It was telling that in the beginning, Claudia could barely do two in a row. By the time we taped the segment, she easily did three sets of 15.

Claudia and I trained for a year, as consistently as her schedule would allow. By the time I weaned Claudia off her chocolates and got her used to a regular routine, her muscles looked sleeker and her strength had doubled.

"I did have a lot of fun," says Claudia, "and after a while, I really started looking forward to exercising with Kathy."

The point is, people would assume, "Well, she's thin—she doesn't have to do anything." But it's not about being skinny; it's about how your body is working, like a humming machine. Thinness is in no way a sign of health. Flexibility, strength, and cardiovascular fitness: those are what's important.

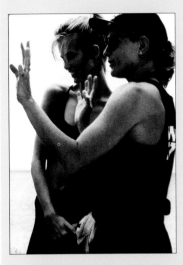

Claudia Schiffer and I

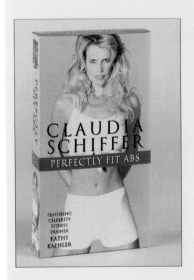

Claudia also felt more energetic and, I think, more confident about what she could do. "The more I started working out, the better I felt about myself," Claudia says now. "Not only was it great to feel my muscles, but I also liked the fact that I was doing something good for myself."

Long-term, this will help Claudia reduce her risk of osteoporosis. While that's a concern for most women, thin women are at higher-than-average risk. To strengthen their bones, I encourage all my female clients to do weight-bearing exercise and get appropriate amounts of calcium. If you can't consistently fit in several servings a day of low-fat dairy products (or other calcium sources such as broccoli or spinach), consider taking a 1,000-milligram calcium supplement.

How Exercise Affects Stress, Mood, and Fatigue

"It's funny; a lot of people would assume exercise makes you tired," says my longtime client and friend Julianne Phillips. "But I actually get more energy from working out. It puts me in a better mood, just all across the board."

Research backs up Julianne's experience. "Some studies done on the effects of exercise on depressive symptoms—feeling tired, feeling sad—show that exercise can really brighten a person's mood," reports psychologist Andrea Dunn.

Not only is there an immediate boost in mood, but "people who are active more frequently seem to have fewer symptoms of negative mood," said Dr. Dunn. In fact, researchers at the Cooper Institute and elsewhere are studying whether exercise can help clinically depressed people. "I think that if we find that exercise is an effective treatment for depression, it will be because you do it consistently over time, just as you would take a medication," she adds.

Sometimes, when you're rushing to meet deadlines or rushing kids around to their various appointments, taking time for exercise seems like a fantasy. But exercise may actually help you most when you're stressed and exhausted. Taking 10 minutes here and there—and honestly, none of us are routinely so busy that we can't do that—can actually increase your productivity.

"It's funny; a lot of people would assume exercise makes you tired," says my longtime client and friend Julianne Phillips. "But I actually get more energy from working out. It puts me in a better mood, just all across the board."

"Sitting around just adds to that 'wiped-out' feeling," Dr. Dunn points out. "A little regular movement can break that cycle of fatigue. Even moderate exercise can reduce stress and its symptoms and help you get more energy and better sleep."

Michelle Pfeiffer says, "Especially when I'm working, people don't understand—they think I'm completely crazy—that I will, on five hours' sleep, lose an hour to get up and work out. But for me, especially if I'm sleep-deprived, if I can get up and work out first thing in the morning, it really energizes me throughout the day. Whereas if I don't, I feel that sleep deprivation much more.

"I can sacrifice a lot of things in my life that I would love to do," she adds. "But I think exercise is the one thing I really can't. I just have so much more energy, and I also think my mind works better."

I find that being physical also opens people up. Even the first time they see me, clients reveal a lot of personal experiences. Penelope Ann Miller, for example, felt comfortable with me right off the bat. We started out doing a lot of hiking. And we never stopped talking. When you're out together for two hours doing something physical, everything comes out.

I've always thought that if I ever decide to change careers, I'll go back to school and become a psychologist. I picture myself meeting clients at the beginning of a fire trail instead of at an office; we'd hike and talk for an hour. People who felt horrible to start would end up ready to face their problems.

Alfre Woodard is someone who gets emotional, physical, and spiritual benefits from exercise. I started working with Alfre when she was doing a *Star Trek* movie. She needed to be stronger for the film's physical demands, but also didn't want to feel self-conscious in that skintight space costume.

Often when I see her around nine in the morning, she's already been out "kicking it" on the beach for an hour with her dog. She wants to greet the world, be out in the fresh air, and do some fast walking. She always tells me she can think about things when she's out walking. If she has an audition or a speaking engagement coming up, she can go through what she's got to do that day. I think it helps her mentally even more than physically.

"When I'm out walking, and I'm not chattering with Kathy, I'm praying," Alfre confides. "As I work my body, I'm using that part of the day to say my prayers.

"When you think about what an amazing thing the body is, it's your responsibility to take it to its potential. The beauty of movement, the joy—it's another way to me of expressing God."

First Steps

When I started training Michelle Pfeiffer, she didn't really have an exercise program. Now exercise is a habit: she's working out five days a week (before her children wake up). When she's on a film, that just means the workouts are at 4:30 A.M. instead of 6:00 A.M.

Most of us will not be that dedicated; you probably don't have to worry about seeing *your* physical imperfections blown up to movie-screen size. But you can get started safely and work up to a routine that feels right for you.

"I HAVEN'T EXERCISED IN AGES!"

You may not have the time or the money to enroll in behavior-skills training classes at the Cooper Institute. But if you did, one of your first tasks would be figuring out your fitness baseline: exactly where you're starting from. "What we have people do, usually in three- or four-hour blocks of time, is monitor their activity on a weekday and a weekend day," says Andrea Dunn. "And then they count up how many hours they spent sitting. For people who aren't regularly active, this can be a pretty shocking experience.

"Everybody's different, of course. But in general, people find that they're spending a lot of work time sitting at their desk: using a computer or spending time on the telephone," Dr. Dunn continues. Instead of strolling down the hall to talk to a co-worker, many people will telephone from their desk.

Once you got over the shock of how much time you spend on your butt, the Cooper staff would ask, "Are there times in your day that you could reduce the amount of time you spend being inactive?"

Kathy's helped me learn to enjoy working out. She really knows what she's doing. She's got a great attitude, and she makes it fun.

—*Penelope Ann Miller*

You know, I used to smoke two packs of cigarettes a day, drink a six-pack of Coke a day—I was the most un-health-conscious person you could find. Really, if I can do it anybody can do it. It's just about starting.

—*Michelle Pfeiffer*

When I start training my new clients, I think many of them assume (or hope) that we aren't going to exercise at our first meeting. But I'll put someone right on the treadmill. Then, I talk to her. That's a great way to check her baseline fitness level and see how much intensity she can tolerate: I watch her breathing and whether she can comfortably respond to my questions. I also ask her to do push-ups and sit-ups, and I test her flexibility. I may also take some measurements.

After about three weeks of workouts, we'll go back and see how much longer she can stay on the treadmill, and how many more reps she can do. This is also very motivating: she can see how her body's working and prove to herself that this effort does pay off.

Most of my new clients haven't been completely inactive. But there are quite a few of them who are close to their ideal weight, but aren't fit. They might play golf or tennis now and then, but they have no regular exercise program in place. They look fine, and probably feel pretty good, but they're just floating by. To me that's like owning a great model car with very low mileage, just sitting in the garage. If you never turn the engine over, and never replace the oil, it may look good, but it's not gonna run great. Your body is the same way.

Samuel L. Jackson fell into this group. He's very tall and lean with a lot of muscle, but very sinewy. I had met him just a few times, when he picked up his wife, LaTanya Richardson, from one of our workouts, or when I went to see her at home. Sam is a quiet and very sweet man. He was feeling tired in the afternoons and lacked flexibility, in part due to not having the right kind of activity. And as we all are, Sam was getting older and was noticing its effects on his body. What he needed was a regular program that incorporated cardio, strength, and flexibility training. LaTanya kept badgering him to make an appointment with me.

One of his passions besides his career is golf, so he plays whenever he's not working on a film. I remember the first time we worked out, Sam was apprehensive that it would affect his score. He teased me: "I better not be sore! This better not ruin my game!"

So I just took that hour and did a very general, basic full-body workout. My goal was to keep it simple, but still help him get a feeling for how his body was doing and

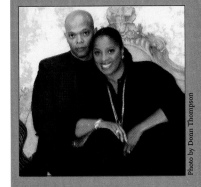

Photo by Donn Thompson

Most days the heaviest exercise I got, other than swimming, was carrying my golf bag.

—*Samuel L. Jackson,
with his wife,
LaTanya Richardson*

what it needed: seeing where he felt some strength, where there might be weakness, and just as important, what moves felt good. At the end, we did a lot of flexibility exercises, stretching his upper back, upper shoulders, and arms. He was not sore. And he came back.

"Kathy told me in the beginning, 'Get on the treadmill and walk really slowly, and we'll build up,' he recalls. "As time went on, I was able to walk a little faster, do a little more, break a sweat quicker...get my body warm, and give it notice: We're about to exercise."

Regular exercise hasn't changed Sam much to look at, but I know he tells LaTanya that he definitely feels better. Gaining a higher level of fitness helps with his golf, as well as his action-film career demands.

SAMUEL L. JACKSON'S ADVICE ON GETTING STARTED

"I'd say to pick something light to begin with. And not to worry about the stiffness or the soreness, because it does go away. I'm a real firm believer in when something starts to hurt, you stop. I don't work through pain. But I will start again once the soreness goes away. And I know it will go away.

"Don't have great expectations of what your physical prowess is anymore. Don't be disappointed when you can't do all the things you think you can do— because your mind tells you you can do things you're not able to do anymore. But with time, you will be able to do them.

"We all want to believe that we're not getting older, we're just getting better. It's an ego thing. But we are getting older. You learn a little patience doing this stuff. You can't overdo it the way you used to when you were young.

"Approach it with some joy, and not like it's a task. View it as fun, and not as something you have to do because you're out of shape, or you want to lose weight. View it as something you're gonna do that's gonna make you feel better. Because you always feel better after you do it."

GOAL-SETTING

The first time I meet with a new client, I start by asking questions: *"Why did you call me?"*

For example, I started working out with Candice Bergen about seven years ago, while she was doing *Murphy Brown*. She called me because she wanted to lose a little bit of weight and get a little more toned. But the greatest benefit she gained was that it helped her relax. She needed that stress-reduction method; it made her feel good.

The next thing I'd ask that client is, *"What is your goal?"* Is it weight loss? Fitting into clothes? A job interview, a movie, a reunion, a sporting event?

About four years ago, I got a call from Maria Shriver. Her third child was about six months old at the time. She'd worked out before, but wanted to try something different; her post-baby body wasn't responding. Her goals were to lose some weight, get back in shape, and have enough stamina to get back to work.

My own goals for a client may not exactly match her starting goals for herself. A potential client may say to me, "I've put on some weight; I've grown out of my clothes and I want to tighten up, flatten my stomach, and lose weight around my hips. I just want to do something for those areas with you in the gym."

What that's telling me is that this person doesn't understand what can realistically be done. In this case, she doesn't realize that there's really no such thing as spot training. No matter how many leg machines you use or sit-ups you do, it's not going to change the fat that lies over those muscles. And I know I'll have a difficult time convincing this person to rethink her goals.

My dream client is one who says, "You know what you're doing. These are my goals. I'm going to do whatever you recommend." This isn't because I'm a control freak. It's because I know exactly what it takes for a body to change, from my education, from training so many clients, and from personal experience.

Once you've read through this book and seen the options available to you, I encourage you to write down your goals, along with the specific steps you'll take to get there. Here's one thing I do personally, and sometimes suggest to clients: carry a little notebook with you and jot down what you think about throughout the day that relates to your body,

> Honestly, it was mainly the way I looked. I wasn't slim, I was just sort of normal, but I felt that pooch around my middle. I wanted to be comfortable with myself, to feel good in clothes.
>
> I didn't have all the energy I used to have; I wasn't sixteen anymore. My knees hurt when I snow-skied. And of course, I wanted to be competitive as an actress. I was in that category where they'll say, "You gotta either lose 10 or gain 40."
>
> —*Peri Gilpin*

all the little things that cross your mind about how you look and how you feel.

Your notebook might contain statements like, "I wish these pants fit me better." "Why can't I lose 10 pounds?" "It's embarrassing to be out of breath after walking two flights of stairs." "I wish I had as much energy as my friend Judy does."

If you're spending a lot of time obsessing about weight or feeling unhappy with yourself, that leads to other goals: reaching a point where you won't be having these negative conversations with yourself, figuring out how you can reprioritize your life to be able to change that. It also helps you pinpoint specific areas where change would mean a lot to you.

Make your goals positive and specific: "By eight at night, I want to still feel as energetic as if I'd had a pot of coffee." "I want to get an A-plus on my yearly physical, including the cardiovascular treadmill test." "I want to sit back and relax by the pool and not think about whether I look fat."

You may have seen that great TV commercial for Special K cereal featuring statements by men that are usually said by women. There's a middle-aged man at a bar, saying, "I have my mother's thighs; I have to accept that."

It's belittling to women in a way to hear a guy say it, but it's so true. Why spend so much time stuck in that ridiculous groove, when you could change if you set priorities and just did it? Wouldn't you like to go through the day without thinking, I've gotta fit in these pants; I really should get to the gym; I shouldn't have eaten that! There's so much more to gain from life.

"How long are you giving yourself to reach that goal?" Of course, everyone wants change to happen overnight. Quick-fix messages blare at us everywhere. But realistic expectations are important to success. Usually 8 to 12 weeks is a fair amount of time to see changes in strength, aerobic capacity, and body composition (less fat, more lean tissue). It can take 6 to 12 months for your body to respond to exercise and to maintain the results. Realize it's not just exercise you're doing; it's a habit that you're forming.

Usually after three months of working with a client, I'll check her progress and reevaluate our goals. One goal I have for Michelle Pfeiffer right now is trying to shave minutes off the time it takes us to run our usual distance.

"Why did you call me?"

"What is your goal?"

"How long are you giving yourself to reach that goal?"

"What have you done in the past?"

"How important is this to you?"

My next question is, *"What have you done in the past?"* That helps me gauge the amount of intensity a client can tolerate and find out about any bad experiences she might have had.

Penelope Ann Miller lives near a popular set of outdoor steps, where hundreds of people converge each morning and evening to get a free workout. I climbed it once with her, and she did it a few times on her own. But each time, she found she had back and knee problems afterward. So we stay away from stairs.

Review which kinds of exercise you might like. If you hate treadmills, for example, don't force yourself to use one. I had one client who'd attended a lot of spinning classes (which use stationary bikes), and was so burned out that she couldn't stand to ride a bike.

Another question I always ask is, *"How important is this to you?"* My view is that being fit should take precedence over everything, because it enhances all of your relationships and everything you do. But I know that not everyone sees it that way. You need to know your own priorities.

Strength, cardio, and flexibility training improve and protect your health while making daily life more comfortable. For example, strength training has given me the confidence that I can go out and walk anywhere I choose. I know I have an underlying amount of strength to handle most things that life demands, while protecting me from injury. I relish the freedom and independence I get from being fit.

Recently, Alfre Woodard surprised her husband, Roderick Spencer, with a gift: workouts with me. "I just turned forty a few weeks ago," he confides. "I wasn't panicking—but you know, my chances of making the Olympic team were getting slimmer! I wanted to get stronger.

"One of the first times we worked out, Kathy said that the true test of strength is how well you handle your own body weight: doing push-ups, pull-ups, and isometrics, not picking up big, heavy objects and putting them down," Roderick adds. These kind of exercises also build agility, balance, and muscle control, as Roderick has noticed at his Saturday morning football game with the guys. He now can last through all four quarters, and his catching has significantly improved.

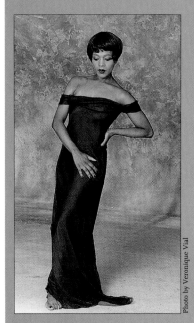

Photo by Veronique Vial

It's hard for me to work out just to look a certain way or fit into a dress. It's got to be more important, or I don't have the heart.

The stamina I get from working out with Kathy... All day long I run up and down the stairs and don't think about it. I can grab and hold my two kids (they weigh 45 and 50 pounds) and put them on my back and run races. I can run and kick a soccer ball for half an hour.

I have practical strength. For me, having a strong body is like owning your own land. I remember the feeling I got when we actually owned our house: "This is mine—you can't come and get me!"

—*Alfre Woodard*

GET OFF TO A WALKING START

Throughout this book, you'll see references to walking for fitness. Why the focus on walking? One reason is that walking is available to pretty much everybody and doesn't require special equipment.

Another is that it's a very safe way to get started with exercise, no matter what your age. Dr. Kenneth Cooper recommends that men over forty and women over fifty go to a physician for a stress test when starting a new exercise program. But he's also realistic. "I know many readers will say, 'I can't afford it,' or 'That's not available,'" he acknowledges. "Then what you should do is limit your exercise program to walking."

If you haven't been moving around much, think really small. "We actually start people off doing two- to five-minute walks several times a day," says Andrea Dunn. "We have them set a very specific goal: 'I'm going to do a two-minute walk at two o'clock, before my coffee break.' If you haven't done anything for a long time, being specific and starting out in small bits is very important." As you feel more comfortable and confident, gradually increase the amount you walk.

So how much walking is enough for fitness? The answer to that question depends on your goals. "If you want to exercise for health and longevity, all you do is exercise by walking two miles in 30 minutes three times a week," says Dr. Cooper. That's similiar to the recommendations in the recent Surgeon General's report: get 30 minutes of moderately intense physical activity most days of the week.

Suppose this is your most important fitness goal (and it's certainly a good goal), but you don't have 30-minute blocks of time free most days? Ten minutes three times a day, even twice a day if that's all you have, will definitely benefit your health and probably lengthen your life (as we described earlier in the book).

What if your current focus is on losing weight? Same plan. A study at the University of Ulster in the U.K. found that short bouts of brisk walking (10 minutes, three times a day) were as effective as one thirty-minute walk per day in taking off pounds.

If your goal is improving your aerobic capacity, on the other hand, the 10 minutes three times a day will help, "but not to the same level that you'd get with 30 minutes of continuous activity," Dr. Cooper adds.

10,000 STEPS TO FITNESS

If you'd like help from modern technology in figuring out how active you are, read on. Andrea Dunn at the Cooper Institute told me about a little device called a step-counter, which they use with their new clients. I have one; it looks like a pager, and you can wear it on your belt like one. It counts every step you take, all day long. How many steps do you think you take in a day?

I wore my new step-counter on two different days. The first day included a three-mile hike with a client, so from 7:00 A.M. to 8:00 P.M. I got in 10,782 steps. Another day, when I zipped by car from house to house, coaching clients through indoor workouts, I recorded only 4,670 steps. (By comparison, my husband logged 7,342 steps.)

"We've done some studies that tell us if people are getting 10,000 steps a day on their step-counters, they're probably meeting the minimum guidelines for physical activity," notes Dr. Dunn. As you can tell from my scores, while it may feel to you that you're always rushing around, if you aren't making it a point to cover two miles–plus on foot you'll never reach 10,000 steps.

"The step-counter gives you your baseline, and then you can set goals to increase by a certain percentage each week," says Dr. Dunn. "We have clients keep track of their steps every day, and we graph their progress so they can see how they've really improved. That's been a great tool for us, because we know that self-monitoring is very important, but it's one thing people don't like to do very much.

"This makes it easy and fun to do. You can look down at your step-counter and say, 'Oh, I've only got 2,000 steps, I'd better try to fit some more in before five o'clock today.'"

The only drawbacks are that the step-counter can't record the level of intensity of your activity or the distance you've gone. If you'd like to try a step-counter, they're available for about $20 from a company called Accusplit in San Jose, California (800–935–1996).

"The goal I have for most women and men is work up to two miles in 30 minutes—
a four-miles-per-hour pace—three times a week. If you want a higher level of fitness,
walk a little faster," he says. "A woman who works up to walking at a 12-minutes-
per-mile pace gets the same cardiovascular benefits as if she were running at a
nine-minutes-per-mile pace, and with fewer injuries."

If you are already doing more exercise than this, don't think you can use this advice
as an excuse to kick back. "This recommendation is for the 48 million Americans at
the bottom 20 percent of fitness, to help them move up," warns Dr. Cooper. "I'm still
running 12 to 15 miles a week, or walking and running because of the Dallas heat.

"But I'm not just exercising for health and longevity," he adds. "I'm exercising
for the quality of life that I want to enjoy, which is quite vigorous. That's skiing in
wintertime, waterskiing and mountain climbing in summertime. I couldn't do what
I'm doing safely—or even do it at all—if I exercised only enough for the health and
longevity benefits."

WHEN SHOULD I EXERCISE?

Some of my clients, like Michelle Pfeiffer, prefer to get exercise out of the way before
they start their day. "Exercise is still for me a chore," says Michelle. "I always have to
make myself exercise, because it's not first on my agenda for things I want to do, you
know? Especially at 5:30 in the morning. But I want to get it done before the kids wake
up, so I can be there for them in the morning."

Penelope Ann Miller is a night owl. "Michelle is probably a morning person and can
wake up early," she says. "I, on the other hand, like to sleep till noon if I can, so I'll
work out more at the end of the day, incorporate it after work instead of before work."

So which way is better? According to Kenneth Cooper, each approach has its benefits.
"The most disciplined exerciser is the early-morning exerciser," he says. "We have
fewer 'dropouts' in the early morning than at any other time."

On the other hand, exercising at the end of the day, before dinner, is physiologically
the best time. "Number one, it burns up the stress of the day," says Dr. Cooper.
"Number two, it suppresses the appetite and helps you control your caloric intake.

Most Americans abuse their bodies by consuming 60 percent of their calories after 6:00 P.M. You sit there, and your body can't handle it."

Then there's benefit number three: late-afternoon or early-evening exercise boosts your metabolism.

"Just check your heart rate," says Dr. Cooper. "You may find, as I do, that your heart rate runs about 48 to 50 beats a minute. I go out and run my two or three miles, and my heart rate goes to 170.

"Now, it comes down rapidly to about 90 in the first five minutes," he continues. "But then it takes two hours to get back to 48 to 50. If I happen to eat during that two-hour period, I have stoked the furnace, my metabolism is higher, and I'm more effectively burning calories."

If you like to exercise in the evening, but can't fit it in until later on, you may be better off sticking to walking. "If I run later at night, because of the endorphin effect of exercise, I come back and I'm wide awake," says Dr. Cooper. "But if I walk a fairly brisk two miles, I then come back, take a shower, and go to bed and sleep all night."

I find that I'm okay exercising at any time of day. When I'm doing my own personal workout, its success depends more on having everything in my life in place so that I can focus. I love to get in a four-mile run at 7:00 A.M., so I don't have to think about it the rest of the day. That also elevates my metabolism, so I might burn more calories throughout the day.

But evenings have also been great for me. Sometimes I'm fried at the end of a stressful day and want to spend time by myself in motion. Sometimes I can most easily work out after the kids are in bed. So make your choice depending on your lifestyle, where you work out, and how or with whom you work out.

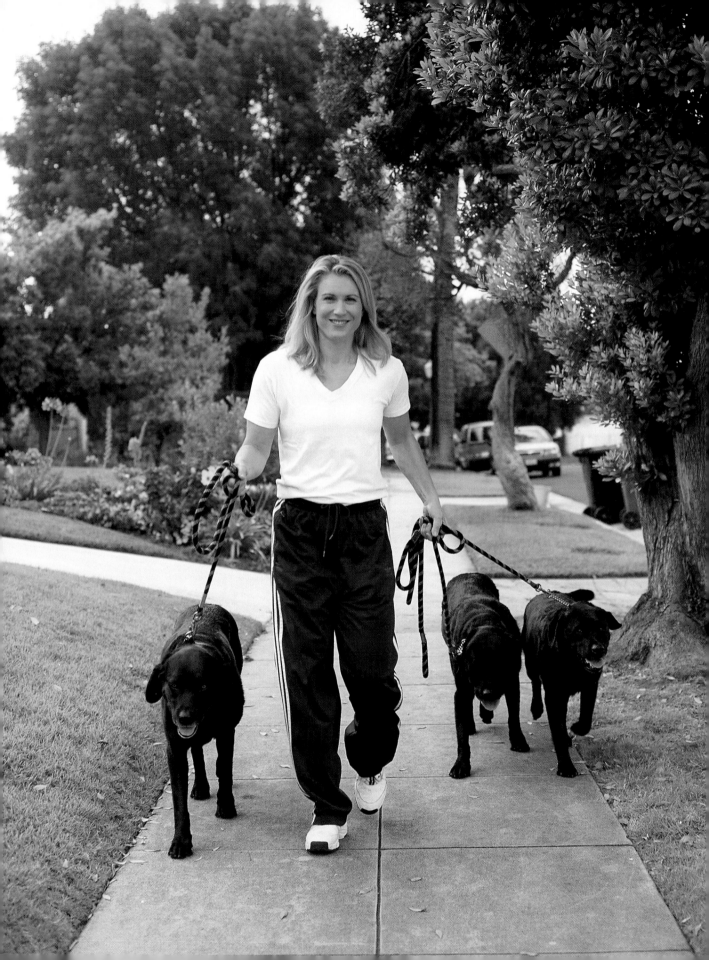

2 STEALTH FITNESS

Sneaking More Activity into Your Daily Life

KNOW PEOPLE WHO EXERCISE ON A REGULAR BASIS; THEY MAKE A COMMITMENT, SACRIFICING OTHER THINGS TO KEEP IT. MY SPORTS AGENT, FOR EXAMPLE, HAS A CRAZY, CRAZY JOB. FROM THE TIME SHE DASHES TO HER OFFICE FROM A BREAKFAST MEETING, HER PHONE'S IN CONSTANT USE: SHE TALKS WHILE HER ASSISTANT TAKES MESSAGES AND SCHEDULES MORE CALLS. SHE MEETS WITH CLIENTS SUCH AS KATARINA WITT AND CARL LEWIS, THEN HEADS OFF TO A DEAL-MAKING LUNCH. THERE ARE ENDORSEMENT PROSPECTS AND MOVIE SCRIPTS TO REVIEW, MORE MEETINGS, OFTEN A COCKTAIL PARTY OR SCREENING. THEN, WHEN IT'S FINALLY TIME TO GO HOME, A CLIENT MAY CALL AND SAY, "I NEED YOU TO FLY TO NEW YORK TOMORROW— WE'VE GOT A NEW PRODUCT."

My agent knows that exercise helps her handle the stress of work—and she tries to fit in early-morning workouts—but her job doesn't allow her to take that hour on a consistent basis. In this section, I'll show you that with some creativity and know-how, it *is* possible to improve your fitness level and shape significantly—no matter what your schedule.

It's important to know that you can break up a workout. If you're a busy person who hasn't been exercising regularly, this is my advice to you: Take 10 minutes in the morning. Go outside and walk around the block. Or, get a jump rope and try to jump for eight one-minute segments, with rest in between. Or, step up and down on a step in your house. While you wait for your child to wake up or get dressed, walk up and down the stairs. Do *something* to get your body going. That 10 minutes of movement *is* worth it.

If you go to an office, you'll have a lunch break. From that hour or half hour, designate 10 minutes to walk around outside or in the workplace. If you're lucky enough to have an exercise facility at your workplace, get on a treadmill or bike—just 10 minutes is okay. You're not going to break out into a huge sweat, and it gives you an energy break. Now you've done 20 minutes of moving.

Near the end of the day, you get home, and you're tired. Let's say you've got kids in the eight-to-fifteen age range. Before (or after) dinner, get everyone in the family to walk briskly around the block, perhaps two or three times. Look—you've put in 30 minutes. And as we saw earlier, that can be as effective as a 30-minute block of exercise—especially compared to doing nothing!

If you followed this advice for a month or two, I'd bet that you'd start to notice, "I've got more energy. I feel more positive, better about myself. I'm getting through the day with a little less stress, less anxiety." That creates that motivation to make exercise a priority. Maybe you'll find yourself getting up 30 minutes early and getting it all done at once. In the following pages, I'll go over a range of ideas for sneaking activity into all parts of your schedule.

"I've got more energy. I feel more positive, better about myself. I'm getting through the day with a little less stress, less anxiety."

Getting Active at Work

You *can* fit in real exercise without giving up your entire lunch hour or returning sweaty to your desk.

TAKE THE STAIRS

"At *Today*, the studio's on one floor and all the support stuff is on the second floor," notes Al Roker. "There's an elevator, but it's very slow. But in the beginning, I used to take the elevator all the time."

I tell my clients, "When you're standing in front of an elevator, ready to go up and down just a few floors, imagine that those elevators do not exist. Or pretend they are broken. Walk away and take the stairs."

"In the last year, I probably haven't taken the elevator more than two or three times," Al says proudly. "I take the stairs, up and down, and that's the way it is."

Consider putting up a reminder sign for yourself and your co-workers. In one study, when cute signs were put up at "choice points" (stairs vs. escalator) in a shopping mall, train station, and bus terminal, use of the stairs more than doubled.

If you often go up and down levels at your job, making stairs a habit can add significant amounts of exercise to your day—and you hardly have to think about it. It's great for your heart. If you work below the tenth floor, there's no excuse not to take the steps.

I've known people who use the office stairs for their workout at the end of the day. They change clothes in their office, go down to the first floor, and start climbing. You could also do some stair-climbing on your coffee breaks or lunch break.

> Kathy sees the possibility of a useful workout everywhere.
> —Alfre Woodard

AT YOUR DESK AND AROUND THE OFFICE

Andrea Dunn has learned a lot of great tips from her clients on sneaking in fitness. "One man spent pretty much all day on the telephone at work, and he didn't need to take notes while talking to people," she reports. "He had a fairly large office, with room to move around. So he got a cordless headset. He had his hands free, and could pace back and forth while he worked."

Another man, a computer engineer, set his computer to beep at him every couple of hours as a signal to take a 10-minute walk. "You have to get a break from the computer anyhow, or you start to get a stiff neck and orthopedic problems," Dr. Dunn points out. "He'd walk a little bit in the morning, walk a bit at lunchtime, and schedule three other little beeps."

"By the end of the day, he'd done almost an hour of moderate-intensity activity, and he didn't even notice it. It was painless."

You might also schedule breaks for some of the exercises I describe in Chapter 3. Take five in the bathroom or break room and do crunches with your feet on the sofa, or do some lunges.

There are also exercises you can do at your desk chair, such as tricep dips, leg extensions, and calf raises. Do pliés while you're on the phone: flip your chair around, and hold on to its back. Put your feet out farther than hip distance apart, with toes pointing at 10:00 and 2:00; bend your knees so they're directly over your toes. Keep your hips slightly tucked under, and your upper body straight. Now, lower yourself down so your hips stay just above your knees. Come back up, and repeat.

This just involves educating yourself about things you can do and committing some to memory. I have an index-card library of exercises in my brain; I know a lot of things you can do with just a chair. So create some mental sticky notes. You don't need a college degree in physical fitness; you just need to know the basic how-tos and know what muscles you're working so you can make balanced choices.

If you get serious about raising your level of fitness, try to get a group of five or six co-workers together. Pool some cash, find a vacant room, and hire a trainer to put you through an aerobics routine twice a week. If you're centrally located and have enough people, it's not that expensive.

OUTSIDE

If there's a pleasant place to walk outside near your workplace, take advantage of it. Walking only requires comfortable shoes. People tell me, "I can't work out during the day because I'll get sweaty, and there's no place to shower." Don't create barriers for yourself. When I walk with clients, we don't get sweaty—unless it's 95 degrees out or we're walking up big hills. Take a mental health break; bring a bag lunch and spend the last few minutes of your break time relaxing and eating your sandwich and fruit.

Stuck-at-Home Fitness

My husband always jokes that he knows if the furniture has stayed in one position for two months, there's about to be a change. I like to turn couches around, move the chairs ... It's not that I'm super-strong, it's just another physical thing you can add to your list.

There are many times when you're at home and you end up doing something that takes 20 or 30 minutes: making a phone call, reading the newspaper, watching a favorite show. And my feeling is, if you are going to spend that amount of time, why not do it while sitting on a stationary bike? You're too busy to get to the gym, so kill two birds with one stone.

"I'm on the phone sometimes for about an hour," says Penelope Ann Miller, "and I end up working out longer on my Lifecycle than I would if I were just sitting there staring into space. If I'm distracted, I don't realize how long I've been working out, and I get a good sweat going. Sometimes I can ride the bike for 45 minutes to an hour while I'm reading a script or watching a video, and not even realize it!"

I remember how I bugged Peri Gilpin to get a recumbent bike, so she could ride while studying her scripts. One day I said, "We're ending our workout early and you're going to buy that bike!" That helps her squeeze more activity into the time I'm not with her.

Other things you can do on the telephone include pliés, and concentration curls with a five-pound hand weight. Do wall sits to tone your glutes and quads while you open your mail.

Try to pay attention to little bits of "down" time you could exploit. When you get up in the morning, do some push-ups off the bed, and some crunches with your feet up on the bed. In the bathroom, sit on the edge of the tub and do some tricep dips. While you're brushing your teeth, you can fit in some lunges and hamstring curls. Take the stairs two at a time, or walk up and down them sideways to work the sides of your thighs. Skim through the body-part exercises later in this book for details on these and others that you could do.

GETTING ACTIVE WITH YOUR KIDS

Suppose you're stuck at home, don't have an exercise bike or treadmill, and don't have a sitter. There's still a lot you can do while the kids are up. For one thing, kids like to copy what you're doing. My cousin would go up and down the stairs at home; her little daughter would go up and down, too. That allowed her to fit in 15 minutes of cardio exercise while her child had fun playing.

To work your outer thighs, make the hose into a loop (tie the feet and waistband together), and put that loop around both calves. Lie on one side, and raise your top leg until the loop is taut. Now, while keeping that loop taut, do 10 to 15 little leg lifts.

Stairs are great for lifts, squats, and lunges to work buttocks, calves, and thighs. (See Chapter 3 for how-tos.)

You can also take two stairs at a time, or hop up the stairs on one foot. Do a stair slalom: standing sideways, jump to the right end of one step, then leap up to the left side of the next, and so on.

The simplest things— sitting on a kitchen chair, getting up, and sitting down— can work as exercise tools. Just repeat 30 times.

Don't overlook the most convenient tool of all—your own body weight. If you can lift your body up and over a bar, come down, and do it again with good form, that's one marker of excellent upper-body strength.

What's important to kids, toddlers and older, is: they want to know you're there. You could sit and watch them play, but you'd be wasting what could be an effective (and fun) time to boost your well-being. One recent afternoon, my kids and I were outside drawing chalk figures on the driveway. They found some little stones and were carrying them from one side of the driveway to the other. I could have pulled out my exercise step, and stepped up and down while enjoying a view of their game. You just have to turn on that mental scanner: I'm going to be out here for a few minutes, so what could I be doing?

Toy pick-up time is another opportunity for a fun family workout. Grab a toy and sprint with it toward the designated storage corner. You can add some squats and lunges for your glutes, quads, and hamstrings. (Make sure everyone has on nonslip footgear.)

Be prepared for moments when exercise can happen. Keep a gym bag in your car containing a sweatshirt, shorts, and tennis shoes. Seeing that bag also serves as a reminder to get active and moving.

Parents are always shuttling their kids around. Many hours are spent in the car, or sitting at soccer games, baseball games, or karate lessons. Those are perfect opportunities to fit in activity of your own.

"One mother I worked with, instead of just sitting with the other parents and watching the soccer game, would walk around the field while her daughter was playing," reports Dr. Andrea Dunn. "She could watch at the same time, yet get her own activity in."

My client Rita Wilson leads a busy life. When we first met, she wanted a fitness plan that would allow her to spend as much of her free time as possible with her kids. One was a toddler; she would put him in a jogger stroller for our runs and walks.

Rita had a small home gym, but her husband, Tom Hanks, was using it to get ready for a movie, and it wouldn't have worked out (sorry about the pun) for her and their child to join him.

Her toddler liked to play with his toys in the driveway. Following my principle of using whatever equipment life makes available to you, I designed a workout for her using these toys. I found a garden hose, a variety of balls (basketball, soccer, baseball), a basketball hoop, a hula hoop, a jump rope, some playing cards, and a wagon. So we

> **K**athy used my kids' toys to create the best workout I've ever done, in my driveway.
>
> —Rita Wilson

did a circuit kind of workout, moving to all the different toy "stations," and got a good cardio and strength workout.

At the garden hose station, I'd stretch out the hose, and Rita would do different kinds of hops and jumps over it: with both feet, on one leg, and then slalom jumps with her feet kept high in the middle. The jump rope station took two or three minutes. Then on to the basketball hoop, where I had her shoot five baskets. The first time, it took ten minutes—and she had to retrieve all stray balls. Her aim eventually improved!

Next was the "card trick" station (see page 66), followed by wagons and balls: I'd pile various balls in the kids' wagons, separate them by about twenty feet, and have her run between the wagons exchanging balls for two minutes. I also had her do lunges up and down the length of her long driveway. Over time, we thought up new stations and mixed them up.

Doing five stations each workout, repeated three or four times, kept Rita's heart rate up for about 45 minutes. We'd finish the workout with some isolation exercises, such as push-ups, a lot of sit-ups, and some stretching—and she had put in 60 minutes without leaving her driveway.

Her son was just starting to walk at that time, so he'd "help" pick up the cards now and then. Mostly, though, he loved seeing his mom running around, playing with his toys. And Rita got a no-hassle workout.

Sometimes after my twins eat dinner, we head out and cruise the neighborhood with our dogs. It's fun for all of us, and when I come back I have a sweat going. If your kids are seven or older, that's a great way for you to be a role model. Issue challenges: "I can make it to that stop sign faster than you!" Then let them set a goal: "This block we walk, the next block we run, the next one we do skipping and two cartwheels." Often kids can be creative when you run out of steam: "Let's leapfrog!" Be silly together. Make some memories.

In the winter, there's walking in the snow, making snowmen, snow angels, snowball fights—how great to get your heart rate up running around the yard dodging snowballs. Watch what your kids do and mimic that.

Be silly together.

Make some memories.

CHEAP BUT GOOD HOME EXERCISE EQUIPMENT

Unless you have joint problems, two-or three-
pound *hand weights* enhance overhead presses,
lateral raises, or tricep extensions, even while
you walk (killing two birds with one stone).
Five- or 10-pound weights are good for
working stronger areas of your body,
such as biceps, while at home.

Ankle weights are helpful for doing leg lifts
and other floor exercises for legs.
If you're already doing twenty-five sets of 4 leg lifts,
weights can take you to the next level.
Don't use ankle weights for walking or doing lunges;
they put too much stress on your knees.

Soft *sandbag weights* add challenge to
floor exercises for lower abs, hips, and rear,
such as pelvic lifts and hip lifts.
You can really feel those extra four or
five pounds on your pelvis.

Jump ropes are another great tool.
My favorite jump rope is called the Animal;
it's about $25 from Super Rope Inc. (414–771–0849).

Many of my clients like to use those big *exercise balls*.
They're sold under many names: physio balls,
flexo balls, workout balls, medicine balls.
I like the ones from the Relax the Back stores;
you can get them from 55 centimeters on up.

HERE ARE JUST TWO OF THE EXERCISES
YOU CAN DO WITH THE BALL:

• For buttocks: Put the ball between your back and a wall,
and slowly "sit," squeeze your butt, and stand up again.

• For upper body: Kneel and rest your torso on the ball.
Hold a couple of soup cans
(or three-pound free weights for you purists)
by your sides and lift to shoulder height as you
squeeze your shoulder blades together.

Use the ball for working outer and inner thighs.
Prop your feet on it for sit-ups. Use it
for push-ups, squats, stretches … you get the picture.
Kids love it, and it's a great conversation piece:
"What's that big ball for?"

Here are suggestions

for inexpensive items

that won't gather dust

in your garage and

will help you achieve a

more vigorous workout.

Being able to keep up with kids is a real motivator. I'm looking forward to doing all this stuff as my twins get older: being outside making forts and climbing hills. There's an indoor gym near where I live featuring gigantic climbing structures, with slides going down. When I get to the top of it, my heart's pounding. I can't wait for those inevitable cries of "C'mon, Mom! Keep up with me!" And having them think they're going to beat me—which will happen eventually!

Sneaking Exercise into Daily Errands

Sneaking exercise into errands may feel silly at first, but it makes mundane chores fun. Carrying groceries (around the store, and into your home) isn't just a chore: it's weight and aerobic training. While putting groceries away, you can at the same time do a set of rhythmic pliés or squats. (Try doing it to music.)

Al Roker advises: "Instead of cruising the mall parking lot for 10 minutes looking for the closest spot to the door, as soon as you pull in, go to the back of the parking lot and walk to the mall. You'll be feeling good about it." In a big city like New York, "Instead of taking a cab, do a combination of walking and taking the subway."

EXERCISING IN TRANSIT

Make time to tighten your abdominals and glutes in your car by doing a pelvic tilt-and-squeeze. Don't recline; keep your seat-back straight up. Rotate your pelvis forward (as if you're trying to look at your belly button). At the same time, contract the buttocks and round your back, so you're pushing your lower back into your seat. (Upper torso stays still.) If you are driving on a city street (not the freeway!), use the time between the lights to hold it; when you stop, release it. You can also do it between stop signs, or do 25 squeezes before the stop. It keeps driving interesting.

If you're on a bus or in a car stuck in traffic, you can do shoulder retractions. Squeeze the blades together, press them back into the seat, and hold, then relax. Do as many as you can. (This reduces tension, and makes you more aware of the back-of-shoulder muscles and upper-back muscles. You don't tend to use these muscles every day, so you lose strength there, affecting your posture.)

You can also do calf raises to give definition to your calves. Stretch your forearms out, and rest them on your thighs. Now raise your heels up so that you're on your toes squeezing your calves, and then come back down. Lean down onto your thighs while you do it to give you resistance. (Women: also read about Kegel exercises on page 110.)

Calf raises are also good when you're waiting outside your car. To do calf raises while standing, just lift yourself up on your toes, then back down again.

EASY OUTDOOR FITNESS

I once did a *Today* segment on gardening: how to make it exercise, and how not to be sore the next day. That started me thinking about all the other things you can do outside. Instead of looking at it as exercise, look at it as activity. The goal is to keep your body mobile and burn more calories. Washing the car is active if you're doing it by yourself: you're reaching up using your arms and sliding down using your legs, and it usually takes at least 15 minutes.

When I lived in Michigan I used to rake leaves every fall. I'd be dripping sweat after picking up those heavy bags and dragging them to the street.

These kinds of purposeful activities are a great way to vary your workout. "I had a little mud slide on my lot during the California rains," recalls Penelope Ann Miller. "My dad, my assistant Monique, and I were out pickaxing, shoveling, and throwing this dirt all over. And I'll tell you, I was sweating like crazy. That in itself was an amazing workout, because we were doing squats and lunges, using our arms and bending over. I was so sore!"

Penelope also found out that her house had beautiful wood floors under the wall-to-wall carpeting. "So we pulled up the rug from the whole upstairs," she says. "We did it all ourselves, pulling it and rolling it, carrying it and hauling it out—plus pulling nails out of the floor. Finding things to do around house, where you're being productive and getting a workout at the same time—that's fun."

Mowing the lawn (especially with an old-fashioned, quiet push mower), shoveling snow, planting, landscaping, chopping wood ... all of these get you moving and give a wonderful feeling of accomplishment. (I recommend stretching when you're done.)

- Raking leaves can be tedious, but the repetitive motion is great for your waistline (obliques and lats). Take this "stealth" exercise seriously—time your session.

- Pushing a shovel and hoe works both arms and midsection. Do it while squatting, and in 30 minutes you've got a planted garden and a good workout. Watering plants and bushes with a hose can take forever; pass the time doing leg extensions for quads and side leg lifts for outer thighs.

- Why spend money on health clubs or car washes when you can have a free car-wash workout? Challenge yourself: allow 8 minutes for a compact or sports car, 10 for a midsize car, and 12 for a sport utility vehicle or truck. That includes drying, windows, and inside cleaning!

PLANNING TO GET ACTIVE

If you'd like a quick list of ideas for fitting the recommended levels of activity into your life, here's one from the *Surgeon General's Report on Physical Activity and Health*. They're listed from "less vigorous, more time" to "more vigorous, less time." (Work up to doing activities like these three to five days a week.)

Washing and waxing a car for 45–60 minutes	Raking leaves for 30 minutes
Washing windows or floors for 45–60 minutes	Walking two miles in 30 minutes
Playing volleyball for 45 minutes	Water aerobics for 30 minutes
Playing touch football for 30–45 minutes	Swimming laps for 20 minutes
Gardening for 30–45 minutes	Wheelchair basketball for 20 minutes
Wheeling self in a wheelchair for 30–40 minutes	Basketball (playing a game) for 15–20 minutes
Walking 1 3/4 miles in 35 minutes	Bicycling four miles in 15 minutes
Basketball (shooting baskets) for 30 minutes	Jumping rope for 15 minutes
Bicycling five miles in 30 minutes	Running 1 1/2 miles in 15 minutes
Dancing fast (social) for 30 minutes	Shoveling snow for 15 minutes
Pushing a stroller 1 1/2 miles in 30 minutes	Stair-walking for 15 minutes

3 "WHAT CAN I DO ABOUT MY...?"

Eight Exercises for Each Part of Your Body

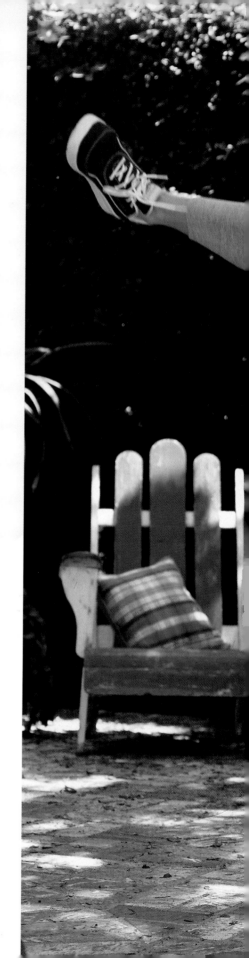

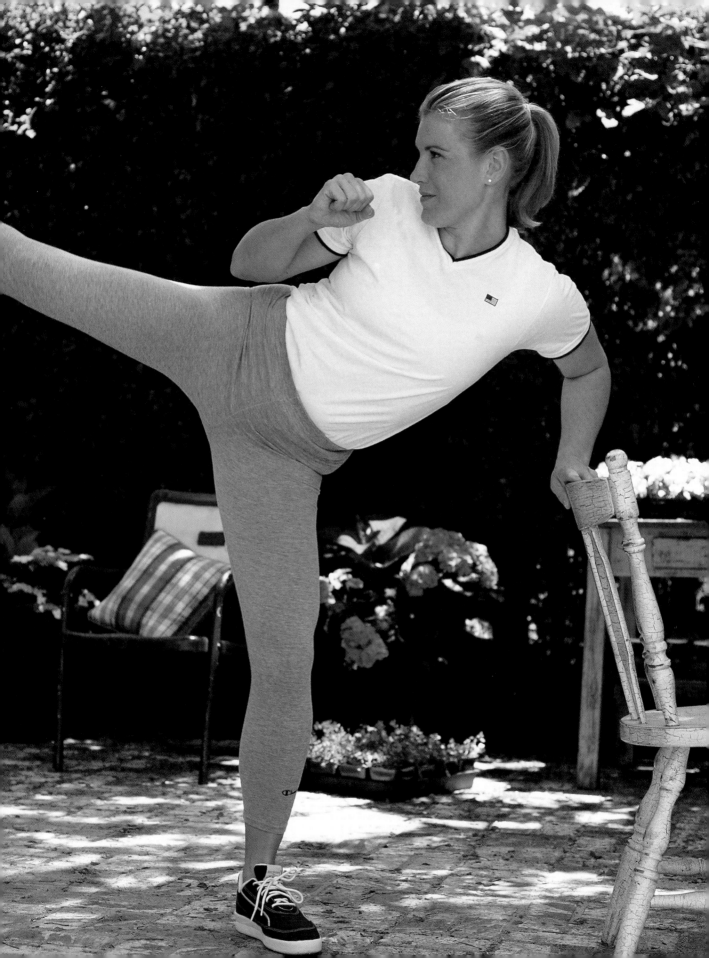

YOU PROBABLY TURNED TO THIS PAGE BECAUSE YOU THINK YOUR STOMACH'S TOO SOFT, OR YOUR HIPS OR REAR ARE TOO ROUNDED, AND YOU'D LIKE A FEW IDEAS ON HOW TO GET MORE TONED AND FIT-LOOKING.

I don't personally know anyone who has exercised from a book. Kinda funny, I know, coming from me. But the books I've flipped through all seem to show exercises you'd do in a gym, and I've never seen anyone in a gym with a book. It's tough to do a bench press while checking a book for what to do next.

I knew of a model who'd buy all the fitness magazines each month, then tear out and pin up all the new exercises she wanted to try. I could see doing that. That's why this section is designed like a menu or an encyclopedia. Skim the exercises and pick out the ones that look fun or are easy to do in the places and times you have available.

I think this chapter will be popular with my clients. For example, I typically work out with Jennifer Aniston two or three times a week. Jennifer always likes to do stuff for legs, so she could check that section to reinforce what we've been doing, or for a new idea or change of pace.

Alfre Woodard can do her own cardio workout (walking or bike-riding), but she often asks me to write down the exercises we do on a piece of paper. This is an example of what I sent to her when she was filming *Down in the Delta*.

Now I won't have to make those diagrams; she can flip through this book and trigger her memory.

REMEMBER TO MONITOR YOUR BREATHING

You'll find it easier if you EXHALE as you START the exercise, and INHALE as you RETURN to start position.

(EXAMPLE: exhale as you raise the weight, inhale as you lower it.)

THINGS YOU MAY NEED:

LIGHTWEIGHT HAND OR ANKLE WEIGHTS

PILLOW

CHAIR

BENCH OR STEP

TOWEL

My Exercise Instructions for Alfre Woodard

Alfre - Do these exercises every other day if you can. Combine this with some type of aerobic exercise.

Get a bike, walk, jog, jump rope etc....

LEGS

lunge 10-15 @ leg

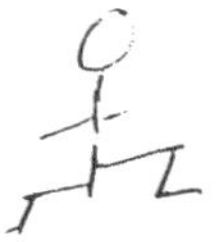

Squat 20 reps.

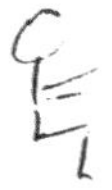

SIDE leg Lift - 30 pulse @ leg ↑ Lift-up

Butt Tucks - 30 w/a weight

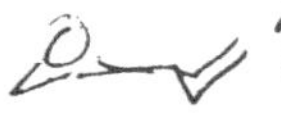

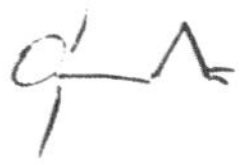

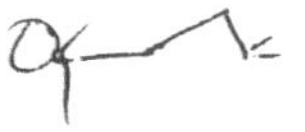

ARMS

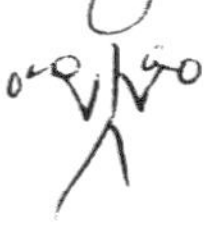

Biceps

3 sets of 15 @ exercise

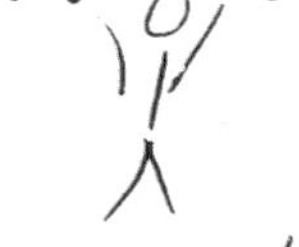

overhead press

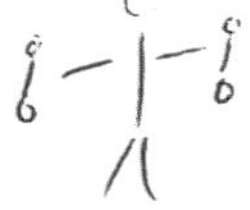

lateral raise

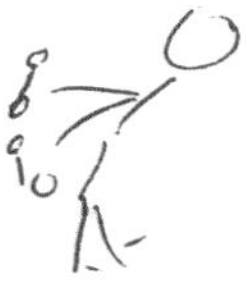

tricep extension

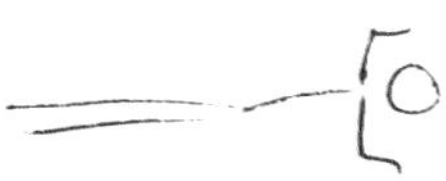

push-ups

ARMS AND UPPER BODY

While not a total upper-body program, these exercises will target problem areas. They'll not only enhance the tone and shape of your arms, but they will help you maintain good posture. If you do these consistently, you'll be ready for those everyday demands (lugging stuff home, carrying a sleeping child) that call for upper-body strength.

SEATED BACK FLY

*For upper back and
back of shoulders*

YOU'LL NEED A CHAIR, PILLOW,
AND HANDWEIGHTS.

*I have Alfre Woodard do this
when we work out because she
gets really tense and tight in
her upper shoulders and neck.
This exercise avoids her neck
area, working the back of her
shoulders and shoulder blades.*

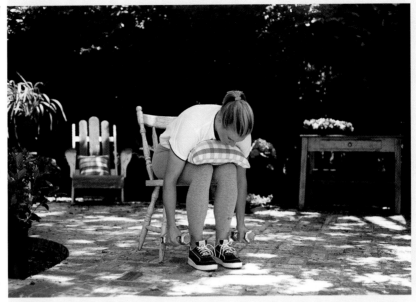

HOW TO

Sit on a chair with a pillow on your lap, arms hanging down, with a three- or five-pound weight in each hand. Now lean forward, resting your chest on the pillow.

Squeeze your shoulder blades together. With elbows slightly bent, slowly raise your arms to the side, going slightly higher than shoulder level. Hold for a beat, then gracefully lower your arms. (Exhale as you lift, and inhale on the way down.)

The key to making this work is to keep your shoulder blades squeezed together (except when your arms are hanging down).

GOAL

Start with 8 or 10 repetitions; work up to 10 or 12, then to 15. If 15 starts to feel easy, it's time to increase the weight (say, from three pounds to five pounds).

BENEFITS

This gives you a toned "bra-strap-area," and improves posture and reduces slouching. It also strengthens your upper back, helping reduce the risk of back pain.

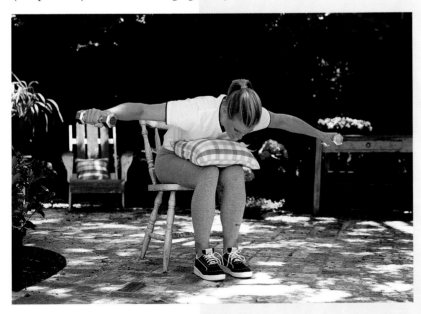

CHEST FLY

For chest and front of shoulders

YOU'LL NEED A PILLOW
AND HANDWEIGHTS.

In her films, Michelle Pfeiffer sometimes wears low-cut costumes, and likes to have some muscle tone there. But like many women, she is weak in her upper body and can't do many push-ups. Sometimes doing push-ups can also cause her to get tight in her neck and upper back. This exercise increases upper-body strength without increasing that tension.

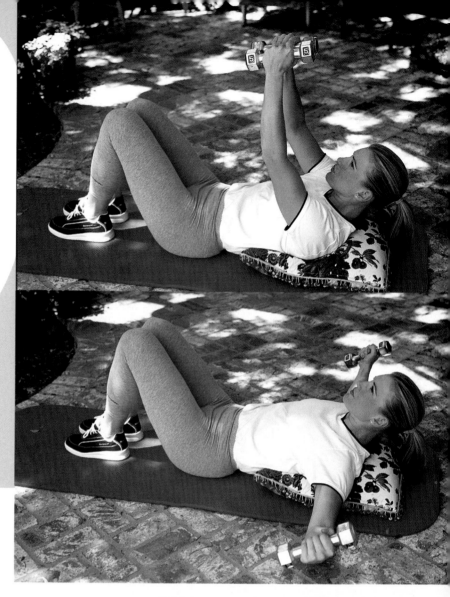

HOW TO

Lie on your back on the floor, with knees bent, feet flat. Place a pillow lengthwise under your shoulders and upper back. Extend your arms straight up—roughly over your chin—with palms facing each other and a weight in each hand. (You can probably use a heavier weight—five to ten pounds—because these muscles are stronger here.)

Slowly lower your arms out to the side, with elbows slightly bent. Keep going until your elbows are just below your shoulders and you feel a stretch across your shoulders and chest. Then bring your arms back up to the starting position. (Inhale as you lower, exhale as you raise.) Imagine you're hugging a giant tree.

GOAL

Try 15. As you improve, increase the weight slightly.

BENEFITS

Realize that this is not about making your breasts bigger: th
no evidence that chest exercises increase breast size. But it
improve the muscles underneath the breasts and give you a
more "lifted" look.

LATERAL RAISE

For shoulders (deltoids)

GRAB SOME HAND WEIGHTS.

Jennifer Aniston is very slight in her upper body. The lateral raise and the front raise (below) add shape to her shoulders, giving a "squarer" look that works better with clothes. Each exercise targets different areas of the shoulder: first the middle, then the front.

HOW TO

Stand with arms at your sides, knees and elbows slightly bent, palms facing in with a three- to five-pound weight in each hand.

Now slowly raise both weights together until your arms are straight out at shoulder level (like a letter "T"). Then lower your arms to your slides. Remember, don't drop your arms: it's slowly up, slowly down. Resist that gravity.

GOAL

This one is harder for women. Start with 8 to 10, and work up to 15.

BENEFITS

This creates shape and tone in your shoulders, which makes your waist look smaller.

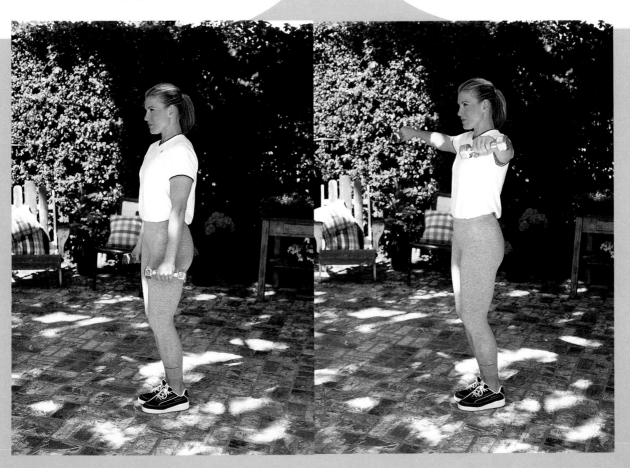

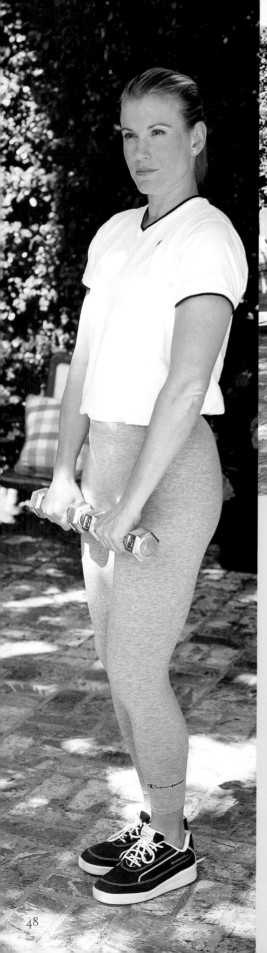

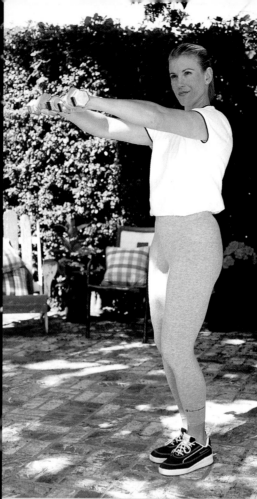

FRONT RAISE

For front of shoulder (deltoids)

USE HAND WEIGHTS.

HOW TO

Start in the same position as above, weights in hands, but with palms facing the front of your thighs. (If a three-pound weight is too much to start, try holding something lighter.) Keep your shoulders back, chest out.

Now, bring both weights forward in a straight line, until your arms are level with your shoulders. (As always, exhale as you lift, inhale as you lower.)

GOAL

This one is also harder for women. Start with 8 to 10, and work up to 15.

BENEFITS

This also shapes and tones your shoulders, and makes your waist look trimmer.

CONCENTRATION CURL

For biceps (front of upper arms)

Because Peri Gilpin's show, Frasier, is regularly nominated for Emmy awards, Peri goes to a fair number of awards shows—and the gowns she wears are usually sleeveless. She likes to have this area toned, so she does the concentration curl and the arm blast (next page) every other time that we work out. These exercises work opposing muscle groups (bicep and tricep). Peri now knows where the muscles are and can isolate them—and she sees progress quickly.

HOW TO

This requires a five- to ten-pound hand weight (one hand at a time). Sit toward the front of your chair, with legs apart. Lean forward and lower the hand holding the weight down between your legs. Rest your elbow or forearm on the inside of your thigh to keep your arm stable. Now curl that arm up, squeeze your bicep, and lower it down again.

GOAL

Start with 15 (your biceps are stronger because you use them daily).

BENEFITS

This reduces arm flabbiness, and gives your arm a more graceful line.

I don't mean to neglect the men; some will want a heavier weight for these. When I work out with Dweezil Zappa, he uses a 30-pound weight for the concentration curl and does fewer repetitions. For the arm blast, he uses a 12- or 15-pound weight.

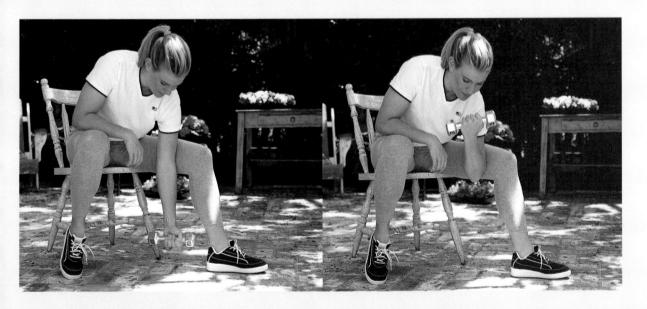

6.7,8

ARM BLAST

Three exercises, using three- to five-pound hand weights—with no rest in between! Do 10 reps each. This is great if you're pressed for time but need to work your arms.

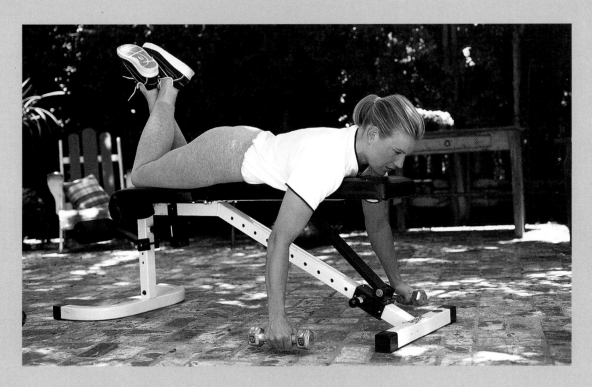

REAR DELT FLY

With arms hanging, lie on your belly on a bench (if you have one) with elbows slightly bent. (If you have a step for step aerobics, rest your middle on that.) Knees are bent, ankles crossed. Your face can be down or to one side.

Now, squeeze your shoulder blades together; raise your arms out to the side (palms facing down) until they're level with your shoulders, then gently lower them.

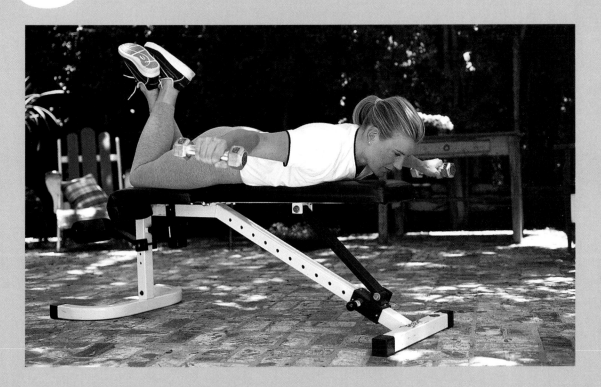

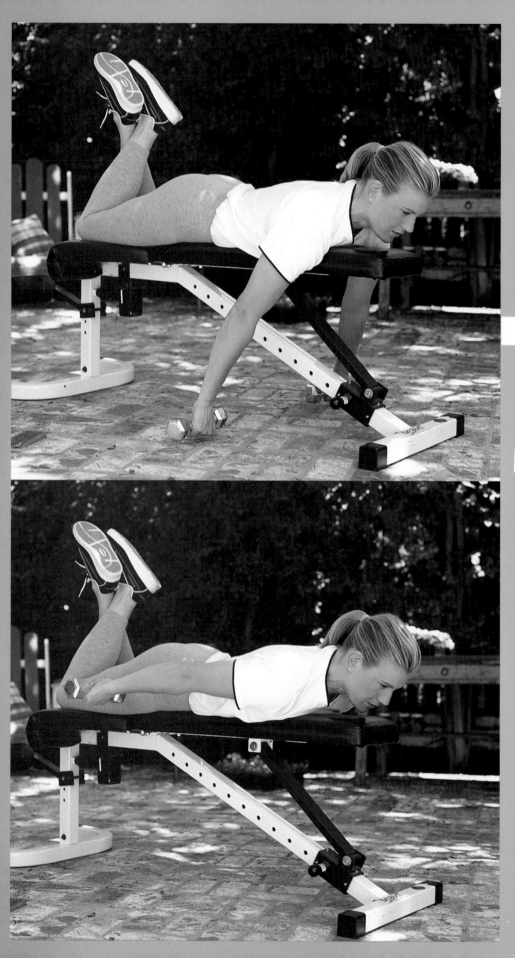

STRAIGHT ARM EXTENSION

Same starting position, except the hand position changes so palms are facing up toward the sky. But instead of lifting your arms out to the side, raise them back, parallel with your hips. Remember to squeeze your shoulder blades and keep your arms straight.

TRICEP EXTENSION

If you like to wear racerback tank tops, this one is for you!

Start in the same position, but bend your elbows so your foreams are up against your ribs. Extend your arms straight, so your palms face your hips, then return to start.

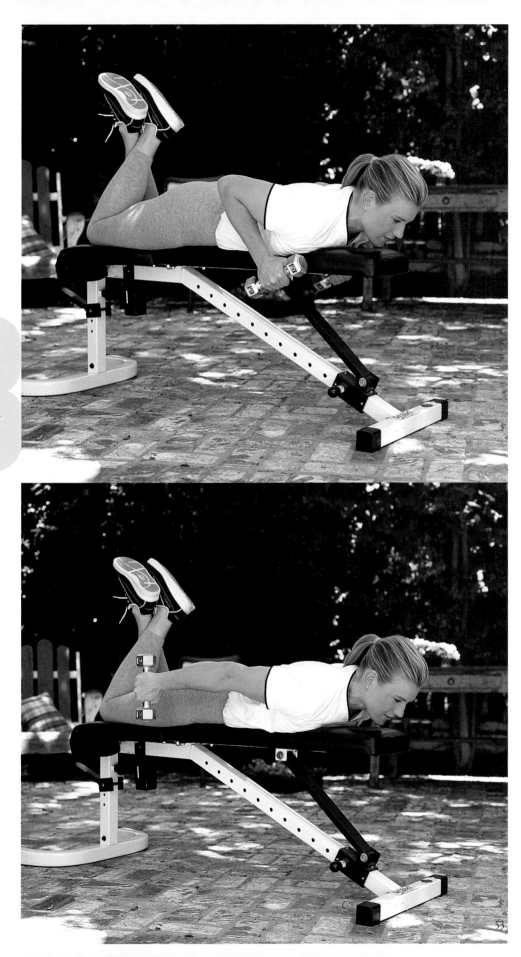

WHAT CAN I DO ABOUT MY...

LEGS

These are classic exercises that have lasted because they're really effective. If done consistently, they will change how your legs look. I use them with all my clients.

I've been doing these with Michelle Pfeiffer for eight years. Since I see her nearly every day, I try to be creative and give her some variety. One day we'll do the four-count leg curl and the knee-up leg lift; the next, it's karate kicks and hamstring curls. If she's feeling stronger, we'll use a heavier weight that day or change the number of repetitions.

Once you have these filed away in your mental Rolodex of exercises, you can do them whenever you have a few minutes (waiting for a phone call, watching television... I'm sure you'll think of many more).

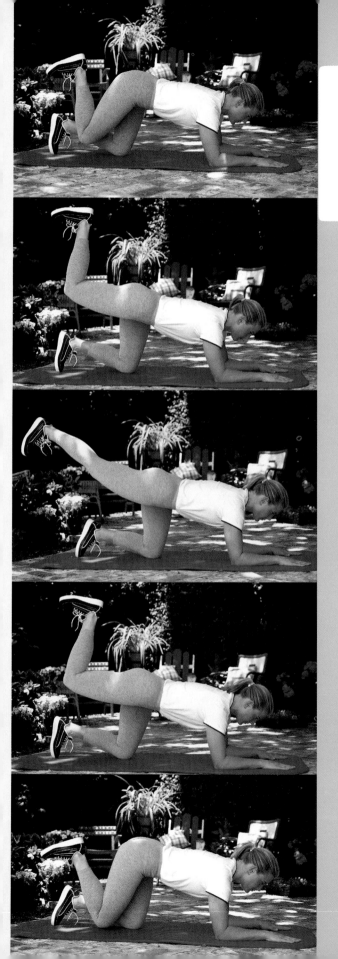

FOUR-COUNT LEG CURL

For hamstrings (back of thigh), quadriceps (front of thigh), and glutes (rear)

YOU CAN DO THIS EXERCISE
WITH OR WITHOUT AN
ANKLE WEIGHT.

Michelle Pfeiffer likes this one because she can isolate those muscles, and feel it working—sometimes feel it too much!

HOW TO

Get down on your elbows and knees, with knees together. Raise right knee slightly.

Count 1: Raise your right knee up to hip level. Foot is flexed. Squeeze and feel it in hamstring and glutes.

Count 2: Point toe and straighten leg.

Count 3: Flex foot again, squeeze hamstring again, bend in your knee.

Count 4: Bring it back down to start. Keep your abs pulled in; don't let your back sag.

GOAL

Do 15 repetitions per leg. If that's too easy, add the ankle weight. Work up to 20–25 repetitions.

BENEFITS

Builds endurance in leg muscles. Good for getting more shape in back of your leg and looking good in shorts.

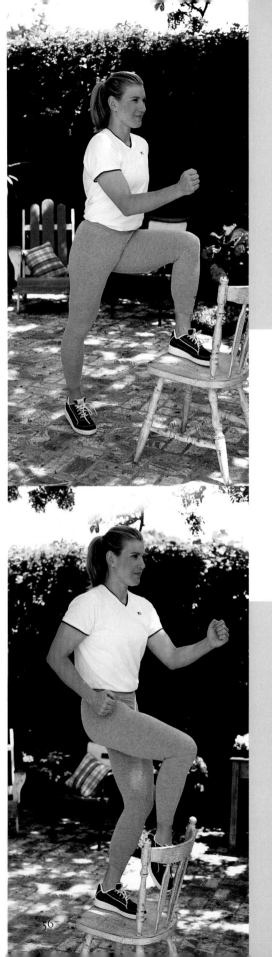

KNEE-UP LEG LIFT

For hamstrings, quads, and glutes

Lisa Kudrow is my lower-body client. She hates to work her upper body (I have to push her) but likes any kind of leg stuff. This one she likes because she really gets her engine going by lifting herself up against gravity.

If you can grab just two minutes while watching your kids play, go for this one, and feel your heart rate fly up like a sprinter's. You'll get instant energy.

Be careful not to simply fling your leg up and down, letting momentum do the work. Concentrate on the muscles you're using. If you can control those movements, you'll work harder and get faster results.

You can do this with a step, weight bench, or sturdy wooden chair (no cushion). If you're new to exercise or have weak knees, use a step (it's lower). If you have trouble with balance, have a partner extend her hands for you to hold as you lift yourself up. For higher intensity, use something higher, but don't use ankle weights here.

HOW TO

Face the chair, with one foot on the seat. With arms out for balance, hoist yourself up, touch the chair with the foot that was on the floor, then come back down—like a giant step-up. You'll feel it right away.

The key is to build momentum, and get your body into a rhythm (but not too fast). To make this more difficult, bypass the chair and bring the knee up and over, toward your chest.

GOAL

5 to 7 reps per leg to start.

Move up to 8 to 10, then 12–15.

BENEFITS

Creates definition in thighs and rear.

You'll feel your heart rate go up, too, which helps burn extra calories.

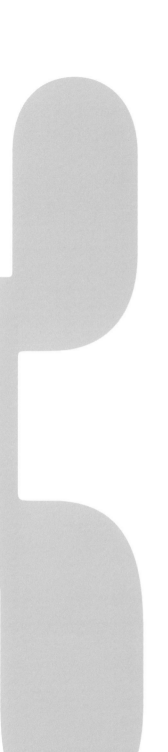

WALL SIT

For hamstrings, quads, and glutes

I suspect that Nancy Travis cusses me out under her breath when I have her do this. But she likes what it does.

THIS ONE REQUIRES A WALL.

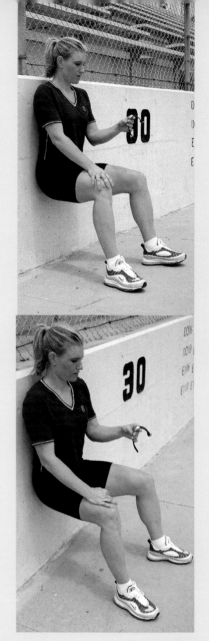

HOW TO

Put your back against the wall. Slide your body down until hips are parallel with your knees. Now hold it as long as you can.

Make sure you've created a right angle with your knee and your ankle, like the side and top of a box. The knee must be directly over the ankle to avoid putting too much pressure on the knee. Hips to head should be a straight line.

To pass the time while doing this one, you can talk on the phone, open mail, look through a magazine, file your nails, hold a baby on your knees— even sing a song.

Stand up when it starts to hurt.

GOAL

Work up to two minutes of wall-sitting.

BENEFITS

Improves strength and endurance in your lower body. Increases muscle density, shape, and tone in legs. Great for skiers.

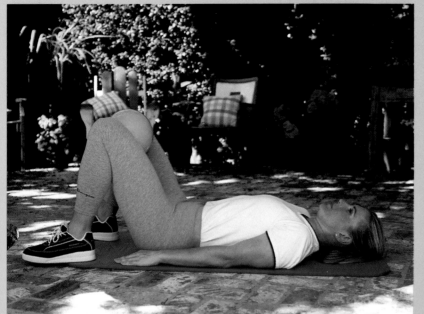

TILT AND SQUEEZE

*For inner thighs,
abs, and glutes*

*Alfre Woodard likes to use
props for variety in her workouts,
and especially enjoys exercising
with a ball. She can do this
easily herself while on location
or vacation. And it's fun.*

4

YOU NEED A MEDIUM-TO-
LARGE BALL FOR THIS ONE:
AN EXERCISE BALL,
BASKETBALL, OR BEACH
BALL WILL DO FINE.

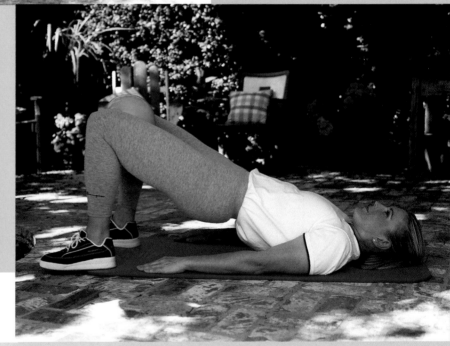

HOW TO

Lie on your back, with your hands at your sides on the floor.
The ball is between your knees.

Tilt your pelvis up, creating a contraction in your abdominals
and pushing your back into the floor. Then return to a relaxed
position. You'll feel this so much it's amazing.

GOAL

Do 10 tilts. At the tenth one: leave yourself tilted, and try to pop
the ball (squeeze hard 10 times—that's the inner-thigh part).
Repeat twice more.

BENEFITS

Tones your inner thighs. And the lower-back stretch feels great.

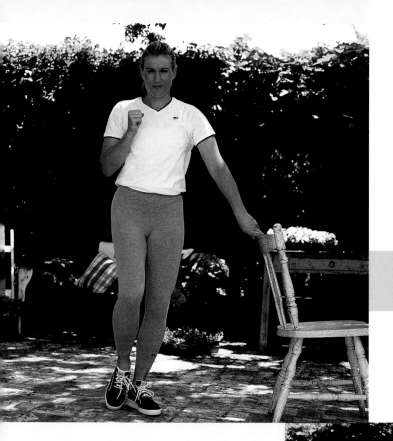

KARATE KICK

*For inner and outer
thighs and waist*

*This is one nice variation
that I do with Michelle
Pfeiffer—it really kicks
up your heart rate.*

You'll need a chair.

HOW TO

Stand sideways to the back of the chair, with one hand
holding on to it. In your mind, just picture what those
guys in the movies do when they do a karate kick. Bend
your supporting leg, and lead with your hip. Kick to the
side and flex your foot. Push your heel up. Do eight kicks
in a row, then turn and do other side.

GOAL

Start with 8 per side. Work up to 10 to 12, then to 15.

BENEFITS

Great for all of your lower body, and helps improve your
balance. Also a strengthener—it takes a lot of muscle to do it.

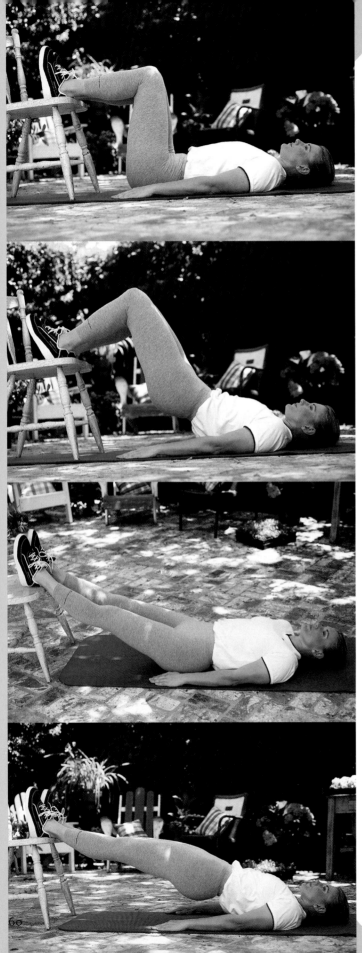

HAMSTRING CURL/HIP LIFT

For glutes and hamstrings (back of thigh)

Lisa Kudrow finds this to be a comfortable and effective exercise. Resting on her back, she can focus on isolating and working backs of thighs and hips.

WITH THE CHAIR AGAIN. (START WITH THE HAMSTRING CURL, AND REPOSITION YOURSELF TO DO THE HIP LIFT.)

HOW TO

For hamstring curl: Lie on your back, hands by sides, knees bent, heels on the seat of the chair. Now press your heels *down* into the chair—not forward—and keep them pressed the whole time. As you lift your hips up off the floor, feel your hamstrings contract. Keep your shoulders and most of your back on the floor. Then bring your hips down again. You'll feel it working.

For hip lift: Legs are straight this time. Push the chair backward. Now, as before, very slowly squeeze your buttocks and lift your body up, so you have a fairly straight line from shoulders to heels.

GOAL

Start with 8 to 10. Build up to 10 to 12, then 15.

Do eight hamstring curls, rest, then move on to the hip lifts.

BENEFITS

An amazing way to target your hamstrings without a machine. Gets your rear and hamstrings toned up like nobody's business.

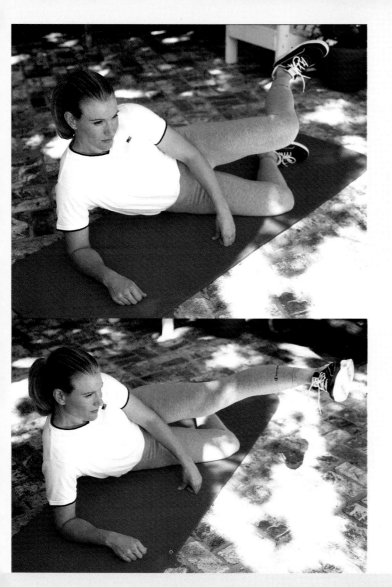

LEG LIFT EXTRAVAGANZA

*A double feature for glutes
and outer thighs*

<small>YOU MAY WANT A MAT OR TOWEL FOR THIS;
USE AN ANKLE WEIGHT FOR MORE CHALLENGE.</small>

*Julianne Phillips has been doing this
combination with me for about seven
years. (We do 45 minutes of step aerobics,
then get on the floor and do our leg lifts,
followed by abs.) You'd think after all
these years we could do a thousand lifts,
but we both still get that burning from
muscle fatigue. Julianne uses an ankle
weight. Leg lifts are fun ... once you're
finished and you know you don't have
to do that side again!*

HOW TO

You'll be doing leg lifts, pulses, repeat, then a kick-out.

Lie on your side on the floor, with knees bent. Your torso
should be in a straight line, with knees coming out from
hips at a right angle.

Be sure hips are stacked on top of each other; don't let
yourself lean back or forward to make it too easy.

First, lift your top knee and leg up without tilting your hip
back, then come back down (don't drop it). Do 10.

Next, instead of 10 counts, do 10 quick pulses, focusing
on the upward motion. Do this 10 times, then repeat the
10 lifts and 10 pulses.

Last part: the kick-out. As you finish the last pulse, don't
bring your knee down. Kick your leg forward 10 times.

Whew!

BENEFITS

This helps the gluteus medius (the upper part of your
rear) and outer thigh. Builds strength and endurance
as well as nicer tone and definition.

WHAT CAN I DO ABOUT MY...

BUTTOCKS

One phrase I've heard over and over again from female clients is, "I gotta work out, I gotta lose weight—and my butt's fallen!" After even a few sessions of doing these exercises, they'll tell me, "My husband has noticed the difference in my rear." Of course, glutes are also a core group of functional muscles, crucial for walking, climbing stairs, riding bikes, and much more.

STANDING LEG LIFT

For glutes (and a little for back of thighs)

GRAB A CHAIR.

Penelope Ann Miller is a big-time dancing fan. She likes this exercise because it has the flavor of dance class.

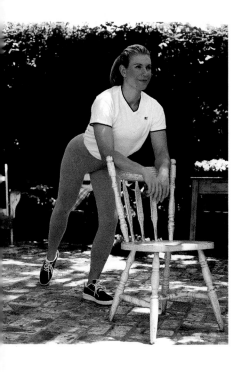

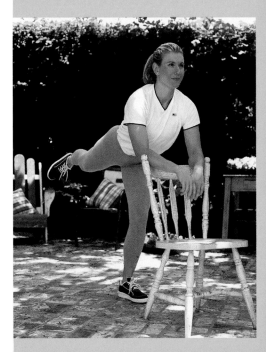

HOW TO

Stand facing the back of the chair, about a foot away.
Lean forward and rest your elbows on the chair. Take
your right leg slightly behind the left, so your heel is
off the floor. Keep your left knee slightly bent. Slowly
lift that leg as high as you can without arching your back.
Hold for a count or two, then come back down again.

GOAL

Do 8 or 10 per leg to start, and build to 12–15.
For more intensity, you can add an ankle weight.

BENEFITS

A great butt, improved muscular endurance and tone,
sculpted thighs, and *strength*. This is great for sports:
skiing or waterskiing, ice-skating, and more.

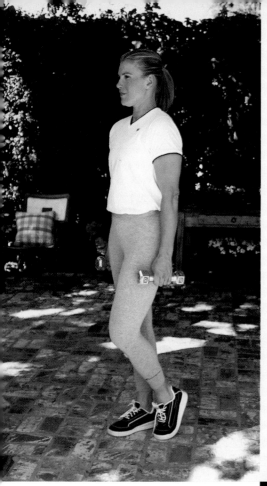

BACK LUNGE

For glutes and quads (front of thighs)

HOW TO

Stand straight, shoulders back, abs pulled in, arms at sides. Take a large step back with your right leg, and bend both knees. Be sure to step back far enough so that your left knee is directly over the left ankle, and your right knee is directly below the right hip (all right angles). To finish, push off and go back to start.

Tip: Keep more of your weight on the front leg. You can increase the intensity by holding three- or five-pound weights.

GOAL

Do 8 to 10 to start; build to 12–15 on each side.

BENEFITS

Keeps knees in the correct position while toning the whole lower body, especially the glutes and quads.

Whenever I do back lunges on Today, Katie Couric always asks, "If people have knee problems doing these, should they avoid it?" Most people sit down and stand up, right? Knees do function in a way that allows back lunges to work. You don't have to be afraid of these, because you just go down as far as you can. Even a little way is effective. I like back lunges better than front lunges because it's simple to find the correct position, and there's no pressure on your knees.

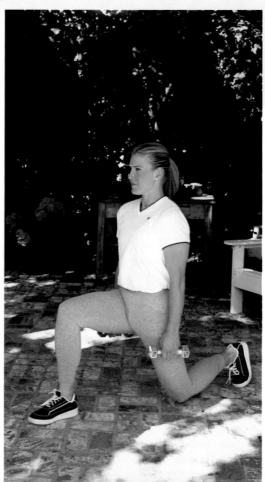

GLUTE RAISE

*For glutes and
back of thighs*

THIS WON'T INJURE YOUR
BACK, BUT YOU MIGHT SKIP
IT IF YOU ALREADY HAVE
BACK TROUBLE.

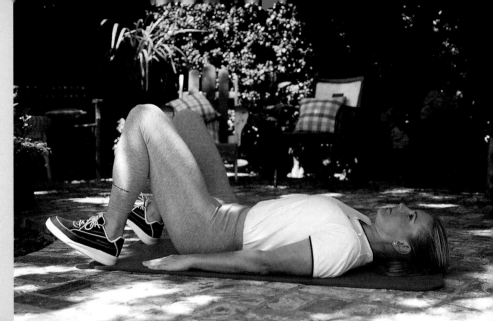

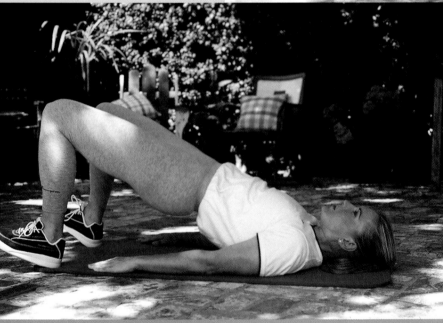

*Nancy Travis likes the glute raise and the glute squeeze (page 68)
because it makes her baby giggle. On her back, on the floor,
Nancy can have the baby next to her or sitting on her hips.*

HOW TO

Lie on your back, feet on floor, knees bent, toes lifted.

Arms are by your sides. Lift your hips and lower back

up off the floor. Squeeze your glutes together as you lift.

The position is similar to the tilt-and-squeeze, except your

toes are up, with heels digging into the floor.

GOAL

Start at 15; work up to 25.

BENEFITS

Helps you concentrate on isolating your glutes from

a comfortable position.

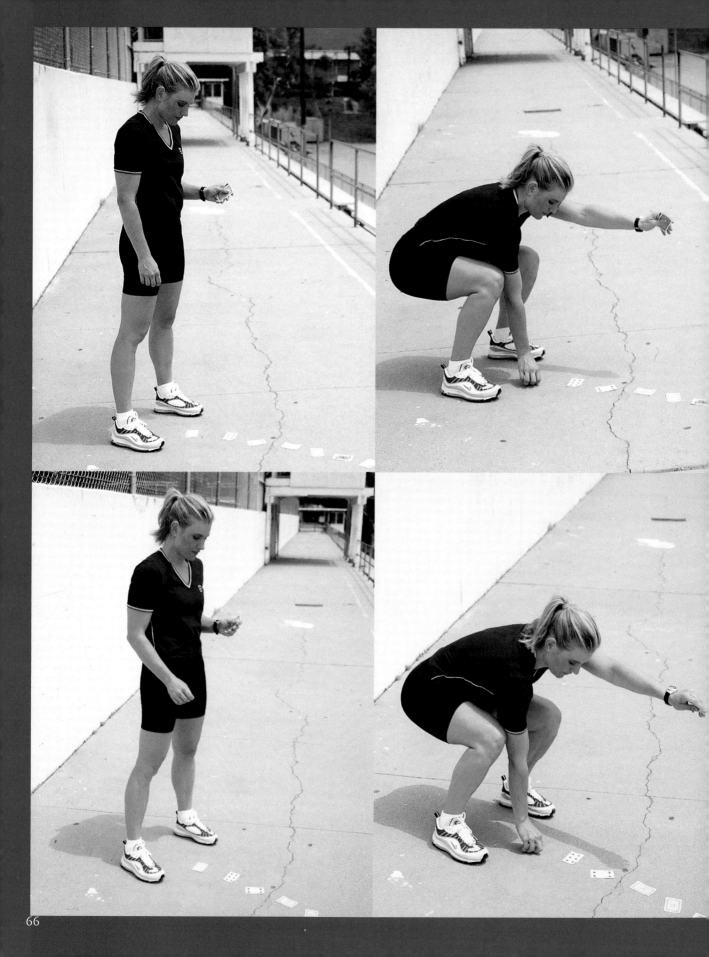

CARD TRICK

For glutes and quads

*I learned this one from fitness trainer Billy Blanks;
I worked with him for four or five weeks to help me
lose that last bit of baby weight. He showed me a
lot of new exercises, and I "adopted" this one.*

*One thing Jennifer Aniston likes about the card trick
is that you can take it with you. She did this in
her hotel room while filming on location in Texas.*

YOU'LL NEED A PACK OF PLAYING CARDS FOR THIS.

HOW TO

Grab 5 to 10 cards. Put the cards in a line on the floor, moving away from you. Stand in front of the first card.

Bend your knees, lowering your buttocks. (Keep back and chest straight, not hunched.) Look for the card with your eyes only—don't dip your head. Pick up the card.

Step forward to the next card. Now, squat down and put the card you've already picked up on top of the new card. Stand up. Squat down again, pick up one of those two piled cards, and stand up. Squat down, and pick up the second.

Now step forward to card three. Repeat the sequence: Put the first card down, second down, so now there's a pile of three. Pick up one, stand and squat, pick up two, and so on.

GOAL

Start with 5 cards, and build up to 10.

BENEFITS

A personal challenge that builds endurance. You'll see great improvement in leg strength and definition, and burn some calories. Easy to do while traveling, and fun!

GLUTE SQUEEZE

For glutes and hamstrings

GRAB A RUBBER BALL
(DODGEBALL SIZE,
OR SIMILAR BALL).

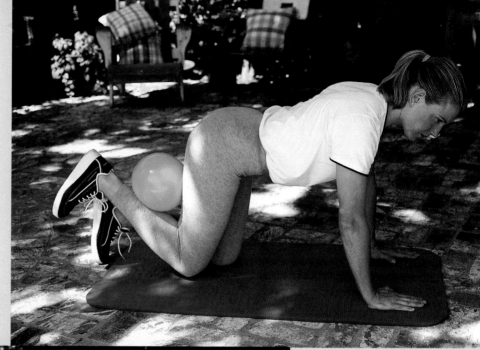

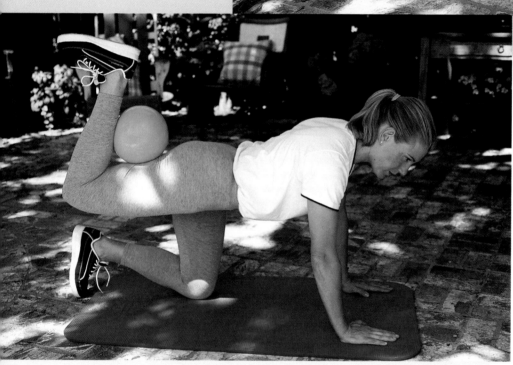

HOW TO

Get on your hands and knees. Hold the ball between one ankle
and the buttock. Now, raise that knee until it's parallel with
your hip. Holding on to the ball, pulse up and down 10 times.
(As you pulse, squeeze your buttocks together, and keep your
abs pulled in.)

GOAL

Do three sets of 10, then repeat on the other side.

BENEFITS

Squeezing the ball contracts the hamstrings, which helps to
isolate them better and work them harder.

ONE-LEGGED SQUAT

For glutes and hamstrings

This is an area that Penelope Ann Miller likes to work; she does it using an exercise step we use for step aerobics. The squat really isolates those lower-body trouble spots.

YOU CAN DO THIS ONE WITH THE TOP OF AN EXERCISE STEP, OR WITH ONE FOOT ON A TELEPHONE BOOK OR STAIR STEP.

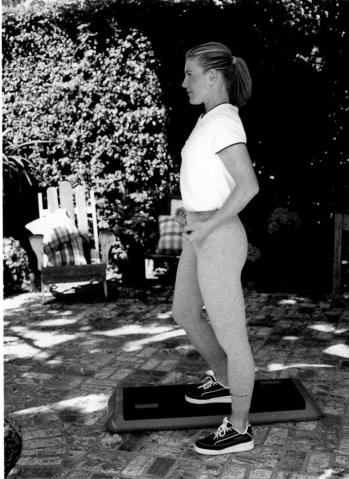

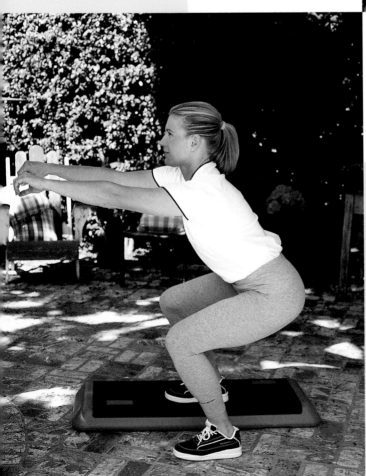

HOW TO

Face sideways to the step. Step up with the right foot, left foot on floor. Feet are hip-distance apart, arms are by sides. Your weight is on the floor foot.

Now, sit back in a squat and reach your arms forward, using arms only for balance. Focus on having your weight rest on the heel of that foot. Come down so your hips are level with your knees, or as far as you can go. Squeeze your buttocks as you come up. Pull your arms in, too.

GOAL

Do 8 to 10 on each side to start, building up to 12–15.

BENEFITS

Lets you work each leg individually, especially if one is weaker than the other.

SIDE LUNGE WITH CARDS

For glutes, quads, and inner thighs

When Lisa Kudrow got a title role in the movie Romy and Michelle's High School Reunion, *Jennifer Aniston gave her my number. Lisa wanted to get fit for the movie, of course, but also to make exercise a more regular part of her life. If time is really tight, Lisa can get away with just this one very effective lower-body exercise. You can do side lunges wherever you are, without a lot of room and equipment.*

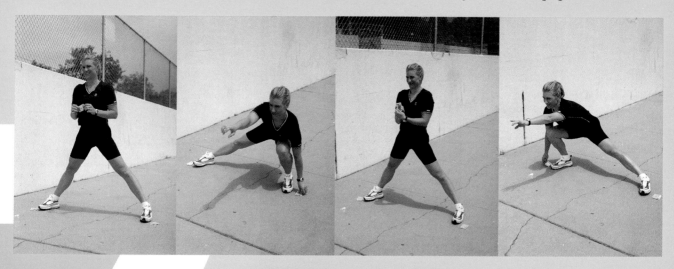

HOW TO

Grab 10 playing cards and place them in a pile next to your right shoe. Stand up, and move your left leg out into a straddle position. You'll be lunging sideways with this one.

Bend your right knee and lower yourself toward the floor, being careful not to hunch your back. With your right hand, pick up one card; extend your left arm in front of you for balance. Then, come back up to the middle, until both legs are straight, and stand.

Move the card to your left hand, repeat the lunge, and put the card down by your left shoe. Stand up. Repeat the right and left pattern, moving one card at a time

GOAL

To get all 10 cards piled on the other side (that's 20 bends up and down). You can work up to 20 cards.

BENEFITS

Builds strength using your own body weight. Helps your ability to isolate muscle groups. Lifts your rear end (especially nice if you're over 35).

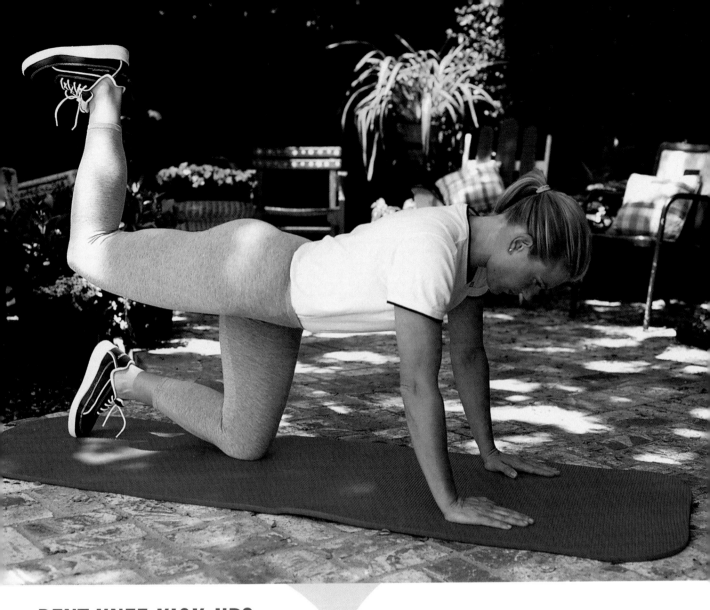

BENT-KNEE KICK-UPS *For glutes and hamstrings*

Michelle Pfeiffer's least-favorite area is her rear, and this really works it. Kick-ups are
a bit more intense than the others in this section because your legs stay in the air longer.

HOW TO

Get down on all fours, on elbows and knees or hands
and knees. Keep your back really straight and your
abdominals pulled in.

Slowly raise one leg off the floor, at a 45-degree angle,
until the knee is level with your hip. As you reach hip
level, contract the muscles in your buttocks and back of
thigh. (Keep your foot flexed—flat and level with the floor.)

Keeping the knee at hip height, pulse leg upward 3 times,
then lower your leg.

GOAL

Start with a set of 5 for each leg, and work up to 10.

BENEFITS

This isolates and lifts your rear. You'll really feel this
working on the back of the thigh. It gives you more
strength for hiking, skiing, and other activities.

71

WHAT CAN I DO ABOUT MY...

ABS

?

Everyone wants a flatter belly. These exercises will also increase your abdominal strength, reduce strain on your back (cutting your risk for back pain), and improve your posture.

OBLIQUE CRUNCHES

For obliques (the sides of your waist)

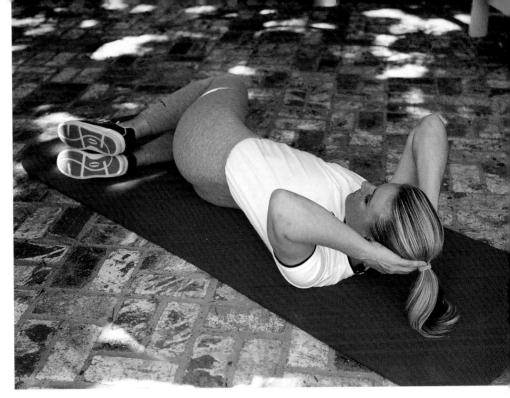

HOW TO

Lie on your back on a mat, towel, or carpet with your hands behind your head. Bend your knees and let your legs fall together to one side—but keep your upper body flat on the floor. Now lift your upper body until your shoulder blades come off the ground—but no farther.

While you're lifting, picture your last rib and your hip bone coming together.

GOAL

Do 8 per side. Move up to 15, and then to 20.

BENEFITS

Oblique crunches give you a firmer waistline; the obliques act like a corset, pulling the waist in.

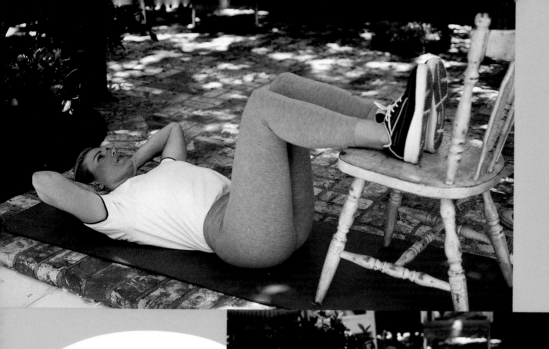

RAISED-LEG CRUNCH

For upper and lower abs

<small>YOU'LL NEED A CHAIR.</small>

Samuel L. Jackson is a back-to-basics exerciser, and this one suits him well. It's effective because the only way you can curl your body up is to contract your abs. The more you do, the more you'll feel it working.

HOW TO

Lie on your back: hands behind head, knees bent, feet up on a chair. (Your thighs and knees should form half a square.)

Lift your upper body, until your shoulder blades come just off the floor. (Don't pull your chin into your chest, or look up over your knees.) Exhale as you come up, inhale as you come back down (this gives you extra energy).

As you get stronger, try it without the chair.

GOAL

Start with 8. Increase to 15, then to 20.

BENEFITS

Along with the other ab exercises, this will give you a smoother-looking belly. But keep in mind: this won't get rid of any fat that's over the muscles. You need cardio (fat-burning) exercises for that.

FROG-LEG CURL-UPS

*Also for upper
and lower abs*

Jennifer Aniston likes these
because that tilt allows her
to feel more of the lower abs.
When she adds the lifting
of her upper body, she really
feels it the whole length of
the central belly muscle.

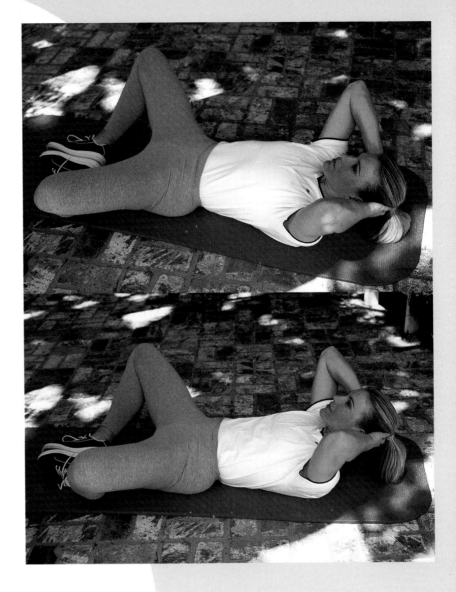

HOW TO

Lie on your back, with knees flopped
apart and soles of feet together (the
classic frog position). Hands are
behind your head.

As before, shoulder blades come off
the floor—but here, tilt your pelvis at
the same time. With pelvis tilted and
shoulders up, hold it for a beat or two—
concentrate on the muscle contraction.
Then, gently lower yourself to the floor.

GOAL

Start with 8. Increase to 15, then to 20.

BENEFITS

This is a variation on crunches, to get
more areas of your abs. You'll feel this
one especially in your lower abs.

KNEE SLIDE

For upper abs

LaTanya Richardson and Alfre Woodard are fans of this one because they both tend to feel stress in the neck. Here, the hand positions allow you to get higher without tightening up through the neck and shoulders.

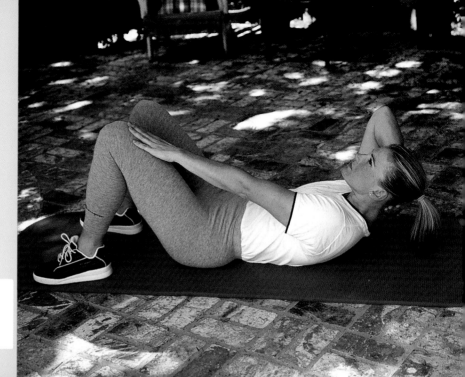

HOW TO

Lie on the floor, on your back, with knees bent. Right hand is behind your head, with left hand resting on your left thigh. Lift your shoulder blades straight up off the floor, and slide your hand up over your knee. Important: keep that hand touching your thigh, because it forces you to push up against something.

GOAL

Start with 8 on each side; work up to 15, then 20.

BENEFITS

The higher you can reach, the better your range of motion.

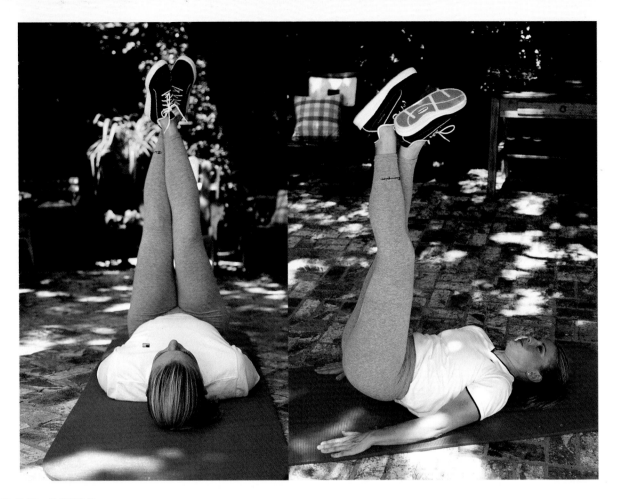

REVERSE CURL *For lower abs*

Awhile ago, I choreographed and appeared in four videos (the Perfectly Fit *series for CBS/Fox) with Claudia Schiffer. We did this one on the abdominals tape.*

I also do reverse curls with Michelle Pfeiffer because she has upper neck and back problems; reverse curls lift only the hips. If you're not strong enough to do crunches comfortably, you might start with these curls.

HOW TO

Lie on your back, arms resting on either side, with palms down. Extend your legs straight up, with ankles crossed. Exhale as you tilt your hips up off the floor—only an inch. You'll feel this working. Then inhale as you lower hips down again. Don't swing or kick your legs—keep them as straight as you can. Don't cheat and push with your hands. As you advance, try keeping your hips off the floor for a beat or two.

GOAL

Do 8, work up to 15, then 20.

BENEFITS

Helps you to learn to isolate your lower abdominal muscles.

CROSS-KNEE
FOUR-COUNT

For upper abs and obliques

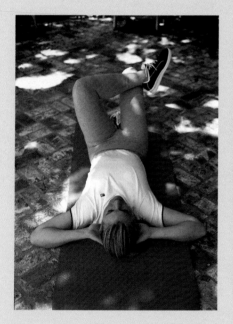 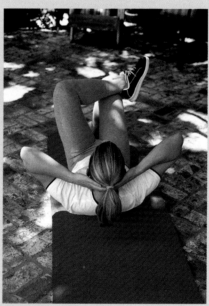 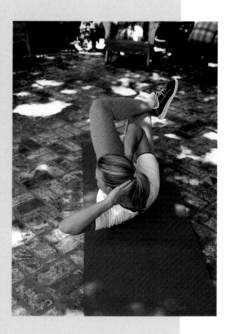

This is an exercise I learned a long
time ago from an aerobics instructor.
I do it with Julianne Phillips, who gets
competitive with me—in a friendly,
motivating way. With the fourth count,
I feel the burn, so I can guarantee
she's feeling it, too. This is a more
challenging exercise because you hold
that contraction longer.

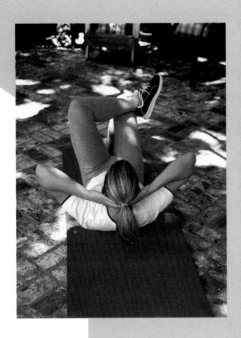

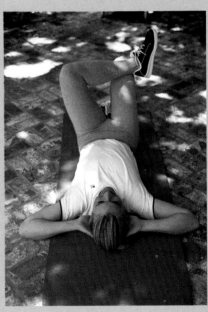

HOW TO

Lie on your back, hands behind your head, left knee crossed with left ankle resting on right thigh. Lift your shoulders up for one count (like a regular crunch), then turn so that your right elbow reaches toward your left knee. Then, without coming down, turn back to the middle. Then slowly come back down. (That's up, turn, straighten, down—four positions. It's the straightening motion that really does it!)

GOAL

Do 5 on each side; work up to 8, then 10.

BENEFITS

Works the abs from all different angles.

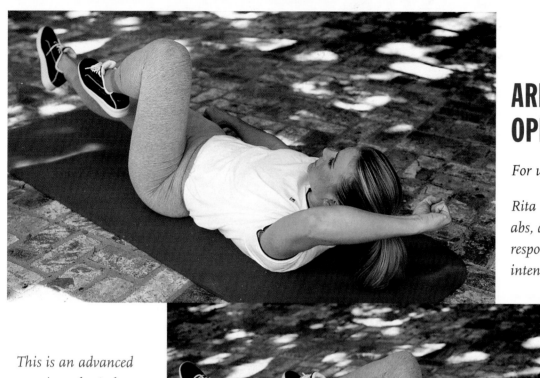

ARM/LEG OPPOSITIONS

For upper and lower abs

Rita Wilson loves to do abs, and she gets a quick response with this more intensive exercise.

This is an advanced exercise—don't do it if you have back problems! It teaches you to go slowly and use muscle control, to actually connect with the muscle. You can't rely on momentum here.

HOW TO

This is an update of the old bicycle exercise, with your arms copying the leg movements.

Get on your back, with right leg straight, left knee pulled up level with your hip, as though you're on a bike. (You can put a rolled-up towel under the small of your back for comfort.) Bend your left arm sideways and over your head, with your right arm pointing toward your feet. (Check the picture; it's tricky.) Now alternate bending and extending arms and legs.

Exhale as you lift your leg and opposite arm; inhale as you place them down. The key is not to do a lot of repetitions, but do to them extremely slowly (as if you're moving through Jell-O).

GOAL

Start with 5, work up to 8.

BENEFITS

This helps with muscle control and coordination. It involves more of your muscles and shows off how strong your abs are getting.

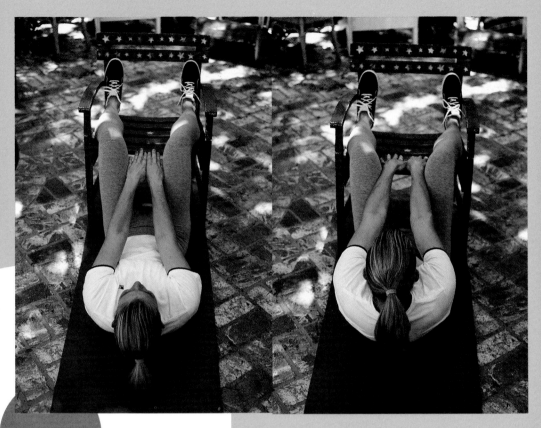

CRUNCH AND REACH

For upper abs

YOU'LL NEED A CHAIR.

I used this to train Rob Lowe when he was filming Frank and Jesse; *it gave him quick results. The crunch-and-reach can be tough because both hands are out there. Your abs must be strong enough to pull you upright correctly, so your head doesn't hang back. Compete with yourself to see how far you can reach your hand on the chair.*

HOW TO

Your back is on the floor, with feet and calves apart and resting on the seat of your chair. Try to rest both hands between your legs, on the seat of the chair. (If you can't, rest one hand on the seat and put the other behind your head.) Reach up and try to slide your hand farther across the seat of the chair.

Focus on how far you can reach. Then slowly come back down.

GOAL

Do eight; increase to 15, then to 20.

BENEFITS

The higher you can reach, the stronger your abs are and the more flexible your back is.

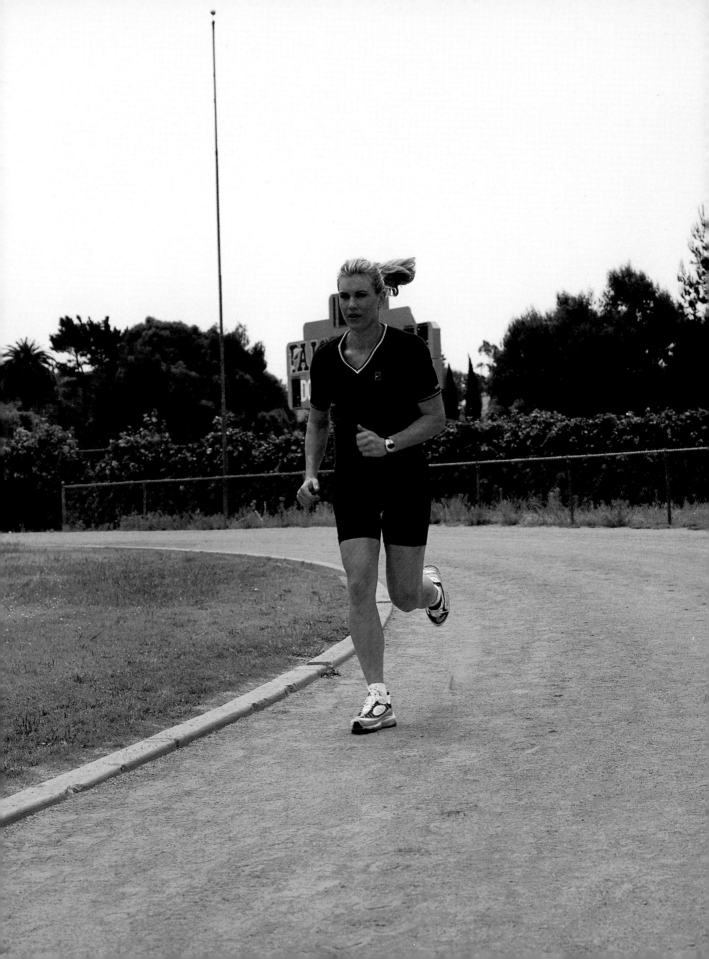

4 EXERCISE FOR OVERALL WEIGHT LOSS

THERE'S NEVER A BETTER TIME THAN NOW TO DO SOMETHING ABOUT THE WAY YOUR BODY LOOKS AND THE WAY YOU FEEL ABOUT IT. BUT THE ONLY WAY YOU'LL GET RESULTS IS TO MAKE IT A PRIORITY.

Exercise physiologist Daniel Kosich talks about what he calls the "if-then" approach to weight management: "*If* I get to a certain weight, *then* I'll finally feel good about myself."

"That immediately signals a negative reality; that person is not happy with herself," says Dr. Kosich. "I try to shift that paradigm, so that the image in the mirror is looked at positively—right now, today."

You're much more likely to succeed at losing weight and getting fit if you can move away from "if-then" thinking. Your attitude needs to be "I like myself right now; that means I'm going to take care of myself."

As Dr. Kosich says, "If you look at eating and exercise from a positive point of view, you'll stay on track. If it's negative, then punishment and self-denial issues creep in. And you probably won't stick with it."

Setting a Weight Loss Goal

Weight loss is simply about energy balance. A calorie is a unit of energy—technically, it's the amount of heat required to raise one gram of water by one degree centigrade. In real life, we use calories to measure our energy intake and output. To lose one pound, you have to create an energy deficit of 3,500 calories: either by burning off those calories with exercise, or by taking in fewer calories when you eat.

"Your body weight, either at maintenance, increase, or decrease, is strictly a function of the relationship of calorie intake to expenditure," says Dr. Kosich. "If you get to a healthy weight and want to stay there, it's critical to eat enough of the right kind of foods most of the time—and to expend an equal number of calories on energy outside, on exercise."

And it's very hard to lose weight when you spend most of your time sitting. Research studies have found that people who exercise to lose weight are less likely to regain it than those who rely on diet change alone.

But how much should you lose? There are a lot of charts and tables out there that tell us what we should weigh. They aren't that useful, however, for setting individual weight goals. For example, the most recent guideline says your body-mass index (BMI), a measure based on dividing your weight (in kilograms) by the square of your height (in meters), should be no more than 25. Formerly, 27 marked the cutoff for carrying excess weight, and a BMI of 30 meant that you were considered obese.

"It's a terrible mistake to try to tell people they're fat and suffering from disease based strictly on height and weight," says Dr. Kenneth Cooper.

"It's a terrible mistake to try to tell people they're fat and suffering from disease based strictly on height and weight," says Dr. Kenneth Cooper. "I would want to have their percentage of body fat determined, because you can be big and lean, or light and fat, and the BMI won't pick that up."

He notes that a football player friend of his was six-feet-six-inches tall, and weighed 290 pounds. "That put him at 33 on the body-mass index, and he has only 10 percent body fat!"

Dr. Cooper points out that it's not only body weight, height, and percentage of body fat that matter: there's also the distribution of body weight. Extra weight around your middle, as opposed to your hips, is more dangerous. "The waist-to-hip ratio in men should be less than 0.85, and in women less than 0.75," he says. "Any waist-hip ratio higher than one is associated with disease. Why do you think the life insurance companies want that ratio?"

A doctor can help you determine these measures, which can be useful in setting goals and monitoring progress. But the most critical weight-management goal is to find a program of moderate eating and activity that you can live with.

"I encourage people to look at it as, What I weigh five years from now isn't determined by what I do for the next week or the next month. It's what I do over the next five years," says Daniel Kosich. "A healthy body weight is the one you're at when you're eating right and getting in adequate activity."

Simple and Consistent

Exercising for weight loss doesn't have to be complex or difficult. Tom Arnold called me when he wanted to lose weight before the opening of the film *True Lies*, in which he co-starred with Arnold Schwarzenegger. As I soon found out, Tom's problem was not a lack of exercise, but the wrong kinds.

He had this enormous weight room, with every piece of equipment a bodybuilder could dream of. But his workouts were primarily muscle burning, not fat-burning. So I said, "If you want to do your weights on your own, or with another trainer, that's fine. We're going to do step aerobics, and I'm going to take you hiking."

We alternated those two, five days a week. When we finished 45 minutes of simple step aerobics, he would have to take off his shirt and wring out the sweat! Then he'd put a clean shirt on and we'd do a little floor work.

After three months of regular exercise, Tom had dropped 60 pounds. Consistency is the key. Even if you work out less intensively than Tom did, you will see results over time if you exercise consistently.

Before I joined *Today*, I had watched Al Roker on the show for a while. When I met him, it was a real pleasure; he's just full of life—charismatic, warm, and friendly. I think with Al, his weight is part of the way he is: it's how America knows and loves him. But fitness

WAIST-TO-HIP RATIO

To calculate your own waist-to-hip ratio, measure your waist at the navel, and your hips at the widest point around the buttocks. Now divide waist size by hip size.

is still an issue for him, as it is for everyone. It was probably two years into my time at *Today* that Al asked me about a place to work out. We talked about exercise, and about what he wanted to do. I had someone whom I was always recommending to people in New York. Al got started at this private gym, and has been going ever since. (Matt Lauer goes there, too.)

"I go at least three days a week; sometimes four," says Al. "One thing that's great about Kathy is that she's not judgmental. The gym's owner, Chris Imbo, knows Kathy, and has the same philosophy: 'It's not how much you do, but that you do it, and on a regular basis.' My weight still fluctuates, but at least I feel far more fit today than I did five years ago."

This past year, Al came out to southern California, where I live, to host the Rose Bowl.

"Every time I tell Kathy, 'I'm gonna be out in L.A.,' she says, 'Call me and we can train together.' And I'd get out there, and of course I wouldn't train," says Al. "In southern California, opportunities for exercise are slim to none: there's nowhere appropriate to walk, because everybody drives out there. So this time, I called Kathy and said, 'You know what? We're training.'"

Al and his wife, ABC's Deborah Roberts, asked me to meet them at their hotel. I had taken my car in for repairs that morning, and I didn't get a ride back. In my mind, this was an opportunity for me to work out, so I jogged and ran the four miles from the car dealer to the hotel. We ended up meeting there twice.

I did what I thought would be good for Al in terms of an overall workout. I wanted to make sure he did some cardio walking, so I had him walking on the treadmill at a fast enough pace so I could see his breathing increase, but so he could still be comfortable enough to carry on a conversation. My goal was to keep him moving to keep his heart rate up, but not do the same thing for a long period, to keep his interest up. We did some treadmill, then bicep curls with light weights, then something for his shoulders, and then back to the treadmill. We moved on to leg extensions, reverse curls to work his lower abs, more treadmill, and then stretching.

This is typical of workouts I do for clients who carry extra weight. When you're overweight, job one is to elevate your heart rate to burn calories overall. I work to find

Al Roker

something aerobic that they can continue for some time. This is often walking. We'll start at 15 minutes and go up gradually to 30 and 45.

If you're quite overweight and can barely walk around the block, start there. Build up to where you can walk around the block twice. Time and again, researchers and fitness experts have found that just walking and building it up over a period of time will cause you to lose weight—and it will come off all over.

"When I can't get to the gym, I try to walk," says Al. "If I travel, I'll do some abs in the hotel room. On the weekends, I like to bike. Exercise has gotten to be a habit; my body expects it."

Maybe you think the effort is not worth it. But it really is—even if you aren't able to lose that much weight. Research clearly shows that you're better off having a body-mass index above 30 (that is, being heavy) and doing regular aerobic exercise than having a BMI of less than 25 and being in that bottom 20 percent of exercisers. As Dr. Kenneth Cooper puts it, "You're better off being fat and fit than skinny and sedentary."

"It's not how much you do, but that you do it, and on a regular basis."

The Body-Part Trap

I've often seen overweight people who say, "Well, I'd like to lose weight but I want to really concentrate on my abs [or arms, or legs]." I'd never say this to them so bluntly, but there's just no point in doing that.

To start, it's more difficult to do a sit-up when you're overweight: you physically can't do it well. It's more effective, and a mental boost, to go out and get challenged with walking and general stretches. You can feel good about doing that, instead of lying on the floor and struggling to do a crunch.

Do exercises that are realistically effective. And once you get some weight off and you can comfortably get on the floor, start slowly. Feel where your stomach muscles are, tighten your middle, then lie back down again. Gradually, you can add more body-part-specific exercises.

Something as simple as getting out there and walking—and really challenging yourself to walk as briskly or as far as you comfortably can—does far more than attempts at a complicated exercise routine. Don't set yourself up for failure by trying to reduce body parts.

Getting Real About Expectations

When I was pregnant with my twins, I gained over 70 pounds, so I've had personal experience with carrying extra weight. (Toward the end, even my tongue felt fat!) When I delivered them, I lost only 18 of those pounds. Now they're almost two years old, and I weigh a smidgen less than I did when I got pregnant. But it has taken me two years.

Putting on weight happens over many months, even years. And it takes that amount of time, or more, to take it off. It's important not to have "program" or "diet" or "that time of year" as the focus for changing yourself. It needs to be, "I'm going to change the way I live, in a way I can live with."

It's important to be realistic about yourself. For me, it's realizing that I'm never going to be the size of Mariah Carey. I'm just not built that way; I have a large frame and big bones. There's nothing I can change about that.

At various times in our lives, we want to be like other people. You have to come to accept that no matter how thin you get, you will not look like that person. Be real about genetics and what you can't change, but also accept that there's a lot that you can. If it's a priority, you'll make changes in your lifestyle so that in time, you can get to a realistic, healthy place for your body. Though this can be hard to accept and hard to wait for, I think people often find that point of view a relief.

Recently I was walking with a client who's in her fifties. Her friend had come with us that day; she goes to Cannes every year. We were talking about women and about life. My client said to her friend, "Are you getting ready for the beach? Getting into your wacky-diet phase?"

"You know, I'm not," her friend answered. "This is the first year that I'm accepting of who I am. I won't waste time trying to look like the 20-year-old bodies on the Cannes beach. I'm going to have fun."

It was refreshing to see someone in L.A. who's not worrying about looking like a 20-year-old. There's really no time to have fun if you always focus on looking right or looking like someone else. That's a tremendous drain on many women's energy.

"I'm happy," she continued. "I walk every day, I eat good food, I have fun with the exercise that I do, and I'm happy with the way I am. I'm finally doing what feels good to me."

We've gotten away from that basic principle because we're so influenced by the media and how celebrities look. It's not about how you "should" look, it's about improving yourself by becoming stronger and more fit. And you have to do it yourself.

Let me tell you a story. Soon after I'd struck out on my own as a personal trainer, I was training an agent who represented one of my actress clients. The agent was overweight; my approach to exercise for her was to do a lower-intensity, longer-duration, low-impact program. We did dance-type aerobics, with simple steps that moved large muscle groups and kept her heart rate up. Usually my sessions last an hour, but since agents' lives are hectic, we were stuck with half hours.

We worked together for six or eight months, and not a lot of change was happening. We talked about this a lot, and I tried to do things to help her move along faster: increasing the intensity, or trying to squeeze in a little more time. I also varied what we did: walking one day, dance aerobics the next, then the stationary bike. I really tried to make this work.

We were already a bit frustrated with each other; she lived in an area that was hard for me to reach during rush hour, and I never knew if I'd be early or late. But the main problem was that she was not changing. One day when I came to work her out, we went into her office instead of our usual workout room. "This isn't working," she said. "I feel I need someone else, and I'd like you to recommend someone to me."

"I completely understand," I said. "I know this is frustrating for you. I wish you could have seen more change, and I'll certainly get someone who, I hope, will have more success."

As I was leaving, I walked past the driveway. And in her car, I saw a giant bag of M&Ms. All this time, she'd been telling me she was eating correctly. Then I thought about how she was saying her lack of progress was because of me.

Since our bodies are mostly water, the amount that you drink or perspire can cause your weight to fluctuate from morning to evening by as much as 10 pounds— depending on your size, of course. And I've talked with Michelle about how the numbers on a scale don't know that you're working out. You will weigh a bit more when you're fit, due to changes in your body composition.

"I think the whole pound thing is really misleading for people," says Michelle. "And if you get up in the morning and your weight isn't what you want it to be, or what you think it should be, it ruins your whole day. So I just go by how my clothes fit. And if the waistband of my pants is a little tight, then I know that I have to watch it for a few days."

Another thing: when a woman reaches her late thirties or forties, there comes a time when she shouldn't focus as much on being thin; it shows in her face, and can actually make her look older than she is. The emphasis has to be fitness: becoming strong and healthy, as opposed to skinny.

And as registered dietitian Michelle Daum pointed out to me, one of the symptoms of an eating disorder is weighing yourself all the time. If you want to have a scale at home, put it in the garage or the basement, so you won't see it in the bathroom every day.

I walked back in and said to her, "I'll still find you someone. But I know I'm giving you quality workouts, and I see another problem. If you want your body to change, you can't snack on M&Ms all the time."

The point is, all of this has to do with oneself. It's not someone else's fault if your body is not changing. You need to do the right things.

Often people will get started, work out, and then go and binge. And they wonder why things aren't moving in the right direction. They can look for someone to blame, but they're just cheating themselves.

If I ask a client to do 15 reps and she stops at five to chat with someone, she's cheating herself. She's not doing exercise for me—I want her to do it for herself. And I can't make her change.

Overcoming Gym Fears

Some people find appearing at gyms intimidating or embarrassing. I've often heard them comment, "I want to lose a little weight first, and then I'll go to the gym." They have to be fit to exercise?

I talk a lot about choices in this book. Going to a gym is one fitness option we have, whether as a regular thing or an occasional change of pace.

"You should not be embarrassed; just go and get started," says Al Roker, who regularly works out at a gym. "The journey of a thousand calories begins with the first step."

"You see these ads for gyms, with these people who are in just incredible shape, all glistening, rippling abs and pectorals—and it's not realistic," Al continues. "I wouldn't want to use the equipment after these oiled-down people have finished with it; you'd just slide off the workbench!"

"But I think people need to get there, and just go," Al says. "Don't worry about the fact that you don't have the right gym clothes, or the perfect shoes or anything. Just go."

It's true that gyms can be strange and uncomfortable places. Even I, a fitness expert, felt intimidated when I first took Penelope Ann Miller to the infamous Gold's Gym. We were surrounded by all this testosterone, and bulging muscles on bodybuilding

> *"Don't worry about the fact that you don't have the right gym clothes, or the perfect shoes or anything. Just go."*

women. I've been inside gyms forever, yet here I was training Penelope and worrying
that I couldn't figure out some of the equipment!

Again, gyms are not at all necessary for getting fit—but they can be useful tools once
you know your way around.

You might also consider hiring a trainer, at least to help get you started on a program.
Not all trainers are expensive. "I'm the type of person who needs the personal trainer,"
admits Matt Lauer. "I think people should try it, whether they pay ten dollars to someone
at the local Y or spend a lot of money for a trainer."

"It's not that I think I'm getting an incredible high-tech workout," says Matt. "The
difference is that for me I feel worse canceling on someone. I feel a responsibility if
I know there's someone who may have dragged herself there just to see me and is
waiting for me."

HERE IS WHAT I LOOK FOR IN A GYM:

First, it has to be convenient. If it's a great gym, but takes half an hour to get to plus parking time, that's a barrier you don't need.

Second, the gym should offer a variety of ways to work out, with lots of different classes (step, low-impact, and aquatic aerobics; spinning; rowing; etc.) and equipment (it doesn't matter what brand). That way, there's a greater chance you'll find things you like and continue to come.

Third, look for a gym that hires instructors and trainers who are certified by the ACE (American College of Exercise) or a similar organization. Often clients don't make use of the gym staff. There should be people around who can discuss your fitness goals, show you how to use the equipment, and give details on classes and programs—and there should be no charge for this introduction to the gym. If you want to use the free weights, most gyms will have a person in that area to assist you in using them properly and safely.

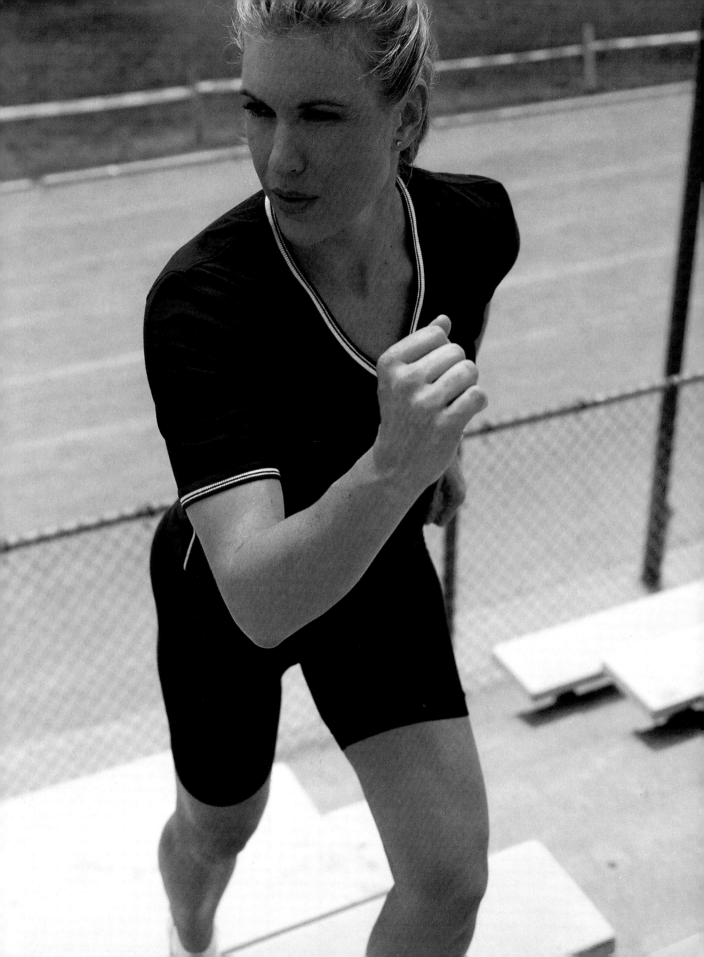

5 EIGHT WEEKS TO A SHOW-OFF BODY

(As seen on Today)

I BET YOU TURNED TO THIS SECTION BECAUSE YOU WANT TO LOOK GOOD FOR SOMETHING SPECIAL: A HIGH SCHOOL OR COLLEGE REUNION, A WEDDING, A BEACH VACATION. IF THE EVENT IS NEXT WEEK, THERE'S NOTHING I CAN DO. BUT IF YOU HAVE MORE TIME, I'LL BE YOUR TRAINER. I CAN HELP YOU FEEL COMFORTABLE SHOWING OFF YOUR BODY.

I first developed this program for *Today*. Both Katie Couric and Susan Dutchers, who develops *Today*'s special series, wanted something to help viewers get ready for swimsuit season. So we sat down and figured out what it would take to get reasonably fast, noticeable results. We came up with a program that can be used by beginners of any age, but is still useful for advanced exercisers. It can also be done almost anywhere— no special equipment needed. All you need are some good walking shoes, a jump rope (optional), and a five-pound hand weight. If you don't want to buy a weight, use a full water bottle. A one-liter bottle weighs about 2.5 pounds.

After the series aired on *Today*, people who followed the program wrote in to tell me about the inches they'd lost. They also saw changes in the tone of their legs and upper body. My eight-week program should also increase strength and endurance. Perhaps best of all, it can give you more energy (no more 4:00 slump), a more positive attitude, and a happier feeling about yourself.

Important: Since this is only an eight-week program, you have to follow it seriously, without skipping. *You need to do it five or six times per week to see real changes.* If you're committed to improving your body, you'll find 30 to 45 minutes a day to fit this in. You might ask a motivated friend or co-worker to do it with you, so you can keep each other on track.

My hope is that if you stick with it, see those good results, and prove to yourself that you have the ability to change, you'll want to keep on finding ways to add activity to your life.

EACH WORKOUT INCLUDES:

a few minutes of warm-up

20 to 30 minutes of aerobic exercise
(burns fat and strengthens heart and lungs)

a short cool-down
(slow down and stretch)

strength training
(also shapes and tones)

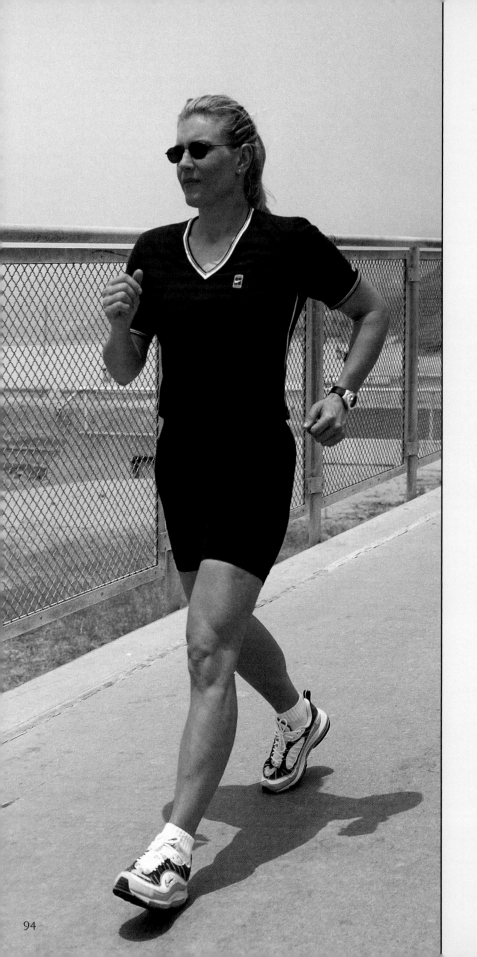

LEVEL 1 WORKOUT

Weeks One and Two

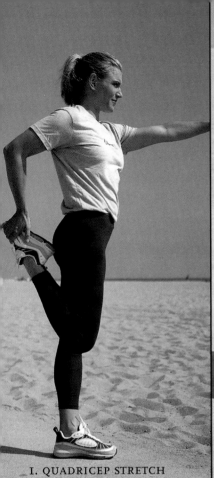

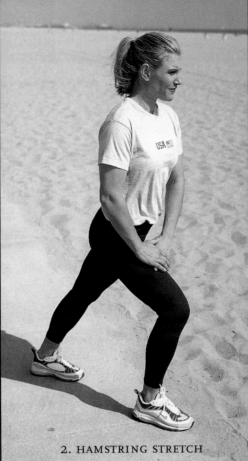

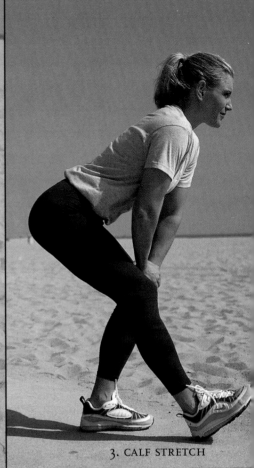

I. QUADRICEP STRETCH   2. HAMSTRING STRETCH   3. CALF STRETCH

WARM-UP

Slow walk (or walk in place)

Start with a slow stroll for 2 or 3 minutes. Once you've warmed up, step up the pace.

AEROBICS

Brisk walk

For these first two weeks, aim for 20 minutes of walking. You're at the right pace when your breathing and heart rate increase, but not so much that you couldn't chat comfortably with a friend. Keep tabs on how far you've gone. Gradually try to increase the distance you can walk in 20 minutes—even by just a half a block.

COOL-DOWN

Slow down and stretch

First, slow your pace and cool off for a minute or two, then stretch. Stretching helps prevent soreness, and it increases flexibility. Hold each stretch for 30 seconds or more—no bouncing. Don't skip this!

I. QUADRICEP STRETCH

(front of thigh)

Stand with feet together. Pull one ankle up toward your hip. Hold the stretch, then switch legs. (Use a chair or wall to balance if you're unsteady.)

2. HAMSTRING STRETCH

(back of thigh)

Bend one knee, then stretch your upper body forward over the other (straight) leg. Hold; switch legs. (You should feel the stretch in the back of your leg.)

3. CALF STRETCH

Stand upright. Step back with a straight leg, and press the back of that heel into the floor. Bend the front knee until you feel the stretch in the straight leg—from the calf down to the Achilles tendon.

STRENGTH TRAINING

1. PUSH-UPS

You can do these the traditional way with your body in a straight line, or with knees bent and ankles crossed and up. (I like to do push-ups off a bench because it increases the range of motion possible. Just lower your chest to the seat of the bench.) Bend your elbows, and slowly move your body toward the floor; then, straighten arms and raise yourself back up. Do 3 to 5.

2. SIT-DOWN SQUATS

You've done this move all your life! Stand in front of a chair, facing away, with arms stretched out in front of you. Slowly bend your knees and sit down, then slowly raise your body back up. Do 5.

3. CRUNCHES

Lie on your back. Bend your knees or put your feet on the edge of a chair. With hands supporting your head, slowly lift your shoulder blades off the floor, and slowly lower them back down. (Do not sit all the way up.) Keep your chin off your chest, and exhale as you lift, inhale on return. Do 10.

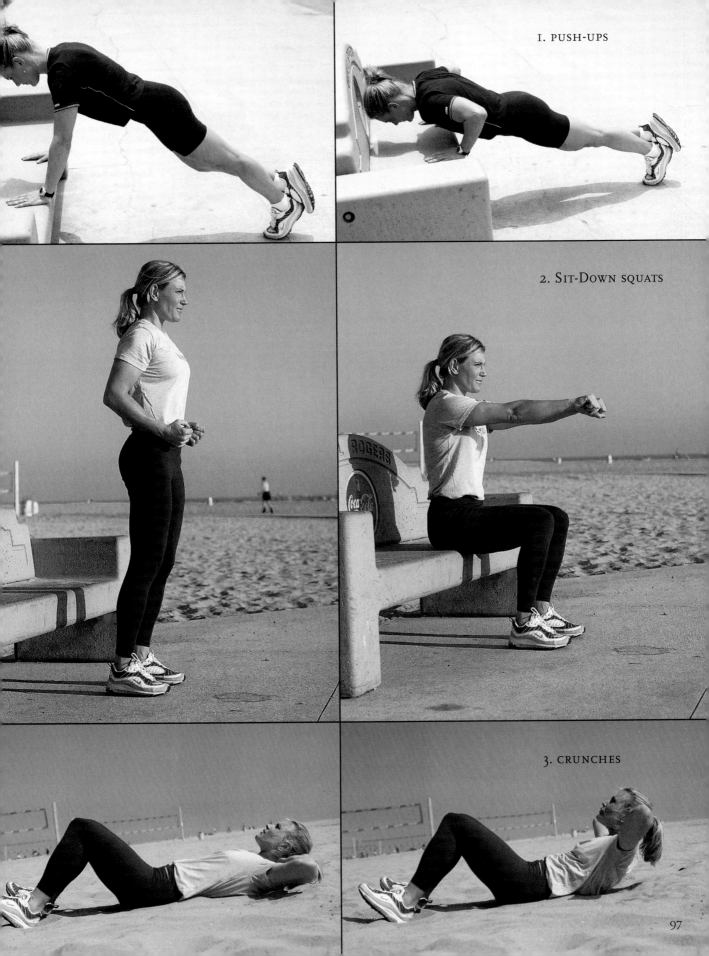

I. PUSH-UPS

2. SIT-DOWN SQUATS

3. CRUNCHES

97

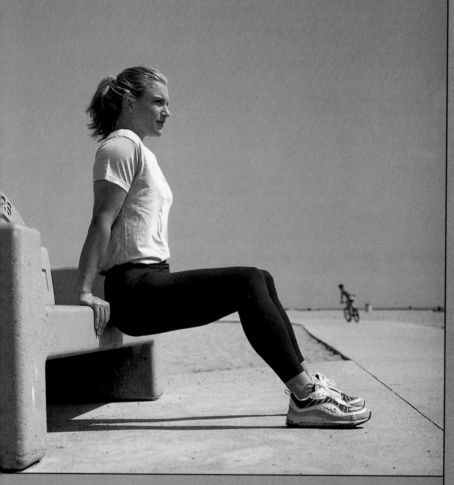

**Weeks Three
and Four**

4. TRICEP DIPS

Whenever I do tricep dips

on Today, *Katie Couric urges,*

"Put your legs out straight—

that's how I do them!" Straight

legs make these tougher.

WARM-UP

Slow walk

AEROBICS

Brisk walk

Move up to *30 minutes* of brisk walking.
Gradually try to increase the distance
you can cover in that amount of time.

COOL-DOWN

Slow down and stretch quadriceps,
hamstrings, and calves (as before).

STRENGTH TRAINING

1. PUSH-UPS
Increase to *5 to 10* repetitions.

2. SIT-DOWN SQUATS
Increase to *20 reps*.

3. CRUNCHES
Increase to *20*. (Flatter abs are
worth the effort.)

4. TRICEP DIPS
(This is new.)

Sit on the edge of a hard chair or
bench, and grab the edge with your
hands. Bending your elbows, dip
your rear down toward the ground
in front of the chair. Straighten your
arms and raise yourself back up.
Keep your back straight and chest
lifted. And keep your body close to
the bench or chair—don't lean
way out to the side. Do 5 to 10.

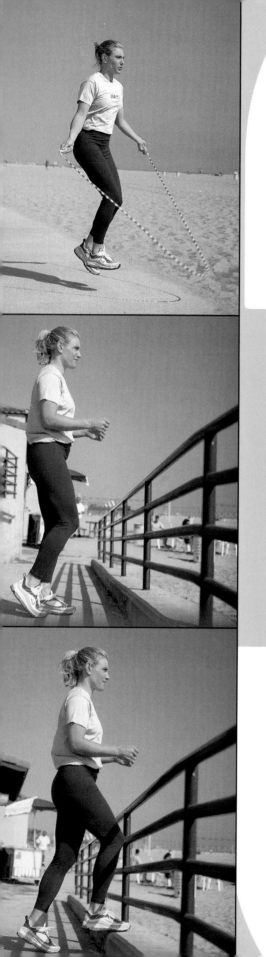

LEVEL 3 WORKOUT

Weeks Five and Six

By now, if you've been faithful, you should see changes in your body—firmer, more defined muscles, and perhaps some inches lost.

WARM-UP

Slow walk

AEROBICS

Add 5 one-minute spurts of more intense aerobic activity to your 30-minute walk. Examples: Walk five minutes, then jump rope for one minute; walk for five minutes, then step up and down on a curb or step for one minute— and repeat five times. (A stopwatch or sports watch is useful here, until you get used to the rhythm.)

COOL-DOWN

Slow down and stretch quadriceps, hamstrings, and calves.

STRENGTH TRAINING

1. **PUSH-UPS**

   You're getting stronger.
   Do two sets of 8.

2. **SIT-DOWN SQUATS**

   Stick with 20 reps, but add a single five-pound weight. Get a chair. Hold the weight with both hands, keeping it in front of your chest. As you sit, push the weight straight out in front (it helps balance you); as you stand, pull the weight back in.

3. **CRUNCHES**

   You need to keep pushing yourself here to make a visible difference in your abdominals. Increase to *two sets of 20*. Make the crunches more challenging by raising your knees, feet off the ground with ankles crossed.

4. **TRICEP DIPS**

   Increase to 12–15 reps.

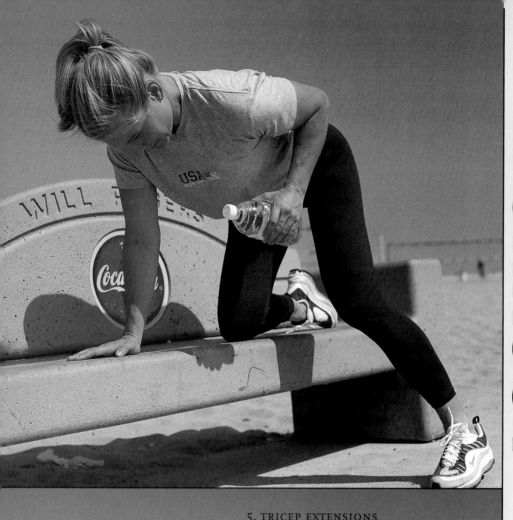

5. TRICEP EXTENSIONS

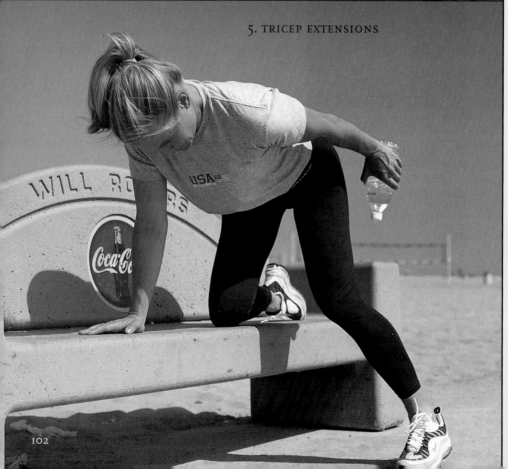

**Weeks Seven
and Eight**

WARM-UP

Slow walk (don't skip this!)

AEROBICS

As before, 30 minutes—alternating five minutes of walking with one-minute high-intensity spurts.

COOL-DOWN

Slow down; stretch quadriceps, hamstrings, and calves.

STRENGTH TRAINING

1. PUSH-UPS

Celebrate your strength!
Increase to *three sets of 8.*

2. SIT-DOWN SQUATS

Increase to *two sets of 20* with the five-pound weight.

3. CRUNCHES

You're making great progress. Increase to *three sets of 25,* with knees up and ankles crossed.

4. TRICEP DIPS

Stay at *12–15 repetitions.* These should be easier now due to the strength you've gained from those push-ups.

5. TRICEP EXTENSIONS

(This is new.)

Facing sideways, rest one knee and hand on a chair or bench. Hold a five-pound weight (or a one-liter, 2.5-pound water bottle) in the opposite hand, with elbow bent and level with your back, against the side of your ribs. Without moving the elbow, extend arm straight back. Then bring back to start. Do 10 on each side.

LEVEL 5 WORKOUT

Week Nine and Beyond

You made it! If you've stuck with me for eight weeks, I know you're looking and feeling good.

By now, I hope your motivation is sky-high, and that working out is becoming a habit. You can continue to build and maintain your strength, cardiovascular capacity, and flexibility with this workout. Along with a healthy diet, this is all you really need to stay in shape.

Schedule time for this routine four to six days a week. If your schedule makes it hard for you to keep setting aside blocks of time, you can break this up. For example, you can walk briskly for 10 minutes in the morning, 10 at lunch, and 10 before dinner.

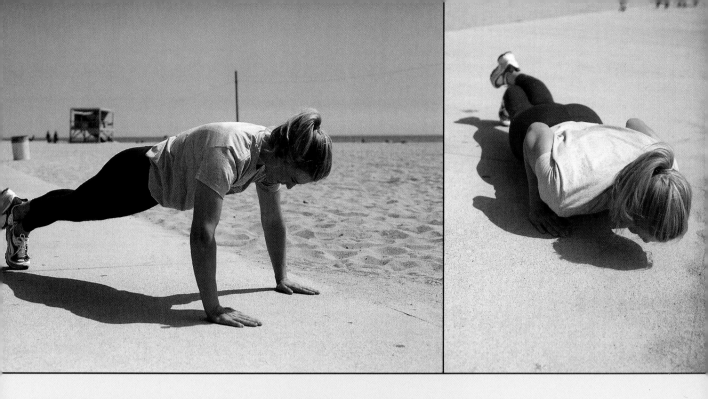

It helps to concentrate on every sit-up, every single rep, and think about how much better you're toning and strengthening the muscles.
—Lisa Kudrow

WARM-UP

Slow walk (or walk in place) for two to three minutes

AEROBICS

Keep to 30 minutes of walking, including five one-minute spurts; gradually increase your speed if you can.

COOL-DOWN

Slow down; stretch quadriceps, hamstrings, and calves. (Hold for at least 30 seconds, and remember not to bounce.)

STRENGTH TRAINING

Do as many repetitions as you comfortably can. As these get easier and you want more challenge, you may gradually increase the repetitions and intensity.

1. PUSH-UPS

Do *three sets of 10*. Variations: Try it with hands farther apart. Or, bring your elbows in so they rub along your ribs—this isolates your triceps (where arms can look flabby).

2. SIT-DOWN SQUATS

Keep this at *two sets of 20*, with a five-pound weight. Variation: Do a set with one heel up; switch heels for the second set. This isolates the glutes (muscles in your rear).

If you want a challenge, do these moves without the chair. Squeeze buttocks together as you stand.

3. CRUNCHES

This stays at *three sets of 25*, with legs up to increase the intensity.

4. TRICEP DIPS

Still at *12–15 reps*. Make them harder by putting your legs out straight.

5. TRICEP EXTENSIONS

Stick with *10 on each side*. I'm proud of you.

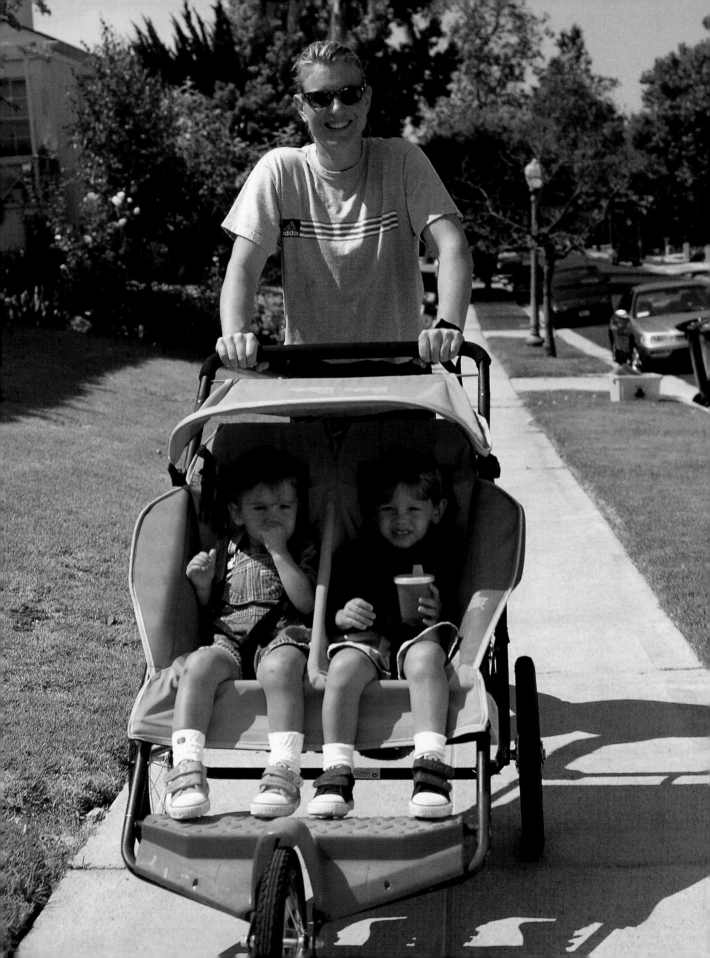

6 SPECIAL SITUATIONS

A FIT PREGNANCY

As in the rest of your life, regular exercise during pregnancy helps you feel and look better. But it also can give you more energy and stamina during labor, and help you get back into shape faster afterward. For example, I had Meg Ryan alternate step aerobics with hiking during her pregnancy. We hiked until the day before her delivery. She had gained less than 25 pounds by the time she delivered. When I saw Meg two weeks later, the pregnancy weight was virtually gone!

The ideal situation is to have an exercise program in place before you get pregnant. You'll be more able to handle the physical stresses of pregnancy. Jami Gertz had terrible nausea at the start of her first pregnancy, and could do only minimal exercise. Before her second pregnancy, we worked out regularly; we ran, hiked, and worked with weights. When she was pregnant, we continued with a lot of walking and light weight training. She had more energy and felt less sick.

If you're already familiar with how your body responds to exercise, this will give you a baseline for comparison as your body changes with pregnancy—which can keep you from overdoing it. I worked out with Michelle Pfeiffer until three weeks before her baby was born. (She was already in good shape from the work we'd done prepregnancy.)

We ran together (but more slowly and not as far as before) until she was three months along, then switched to a combination of running and walking during her fourth month: walking five minutes, then jogging five minutes. One day she told me, "This is uncomfortable. I could still do it, but my body is telling me to do something else." So we tapered off into walking, stretching, and Kegels until she had the baby.

Listen to your body's signals and don't do more than feels right to you. You still can do quite a bit of exercise, and different types, but at a lower intensity. When you're not pregnant, at times you might be really tired but keep pushing yourself. When you're pregnant, listen to your body.

I've found with pregnant clients I've trained, as well as during my own pregnancy, that the best choices are walking or any type of aquatic program. Walking is good because

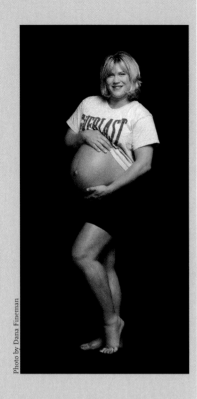

I loved watching Kathy on *Today* gain the weight with the children, then have the babies, and stay healthy throughout that. She's so down-to-earth. And then after the babies were born, she slowly and in a very healthy way came back down.

I thought that was really important, that we could see her twice a month on *Today*, doing this in a healthy way, and not freaking out that she'd gained some weight with her children.

—*Peri Gilpin*

you can do it anywhere, and it puts less pressure on your joints due to lower impact. Swimming's even better because of the buoyancy; it takes pressure off your back and can reduce any swelling you have. I swam nearly every day from my sixth month on, and it felt great. I'd take 10 or 15 minutes and do side scissor kicks from one side of the pool to the other, or kick my legs while holding a kickboard. Then I'd enjoy floating (like a whale) for a while; it was the only time I felt light.

One of my favorite exercises for pregnancy is the "accordion." It's for your belly, and helps strengthen and prevent splitting of your central abdominal muscle. It also reduces back stress, and improves your breathing.

Stand with knees slightly bent, pelvis tilted forward. Imagine you have an accordion in your belly, with one handle against your spine and the other against your abdomen. Take a deep breath and fully expand the accordion. Then exhale partway, so the accordion is halfway closed. (Now comes the real work.) Do small, rhythmic exhales until all the air is out and the accordion is fully closed. Count each of these mini-exhales as one repetition. Do 25 one after the other. (If you'd like more detail on this and other exercises, see my book *Primetime Pregnancy,* listed at the end of this book.)

New-Parent Fitness

"For me, getting pregnant was a go-ahead to eat whatever I wanted. It was the perfect excuse," my client Nancy Travis says. "It was, 'I'm not overweight, I'm pregnant, so I can glory in the way I look.' But six months after the baby came out, I still looked like I was pregnant."

There are some fortunate women, such as Meg Ryan, who quickly lose the weight after pregnancy. They're fitting into their old jeans a few weeks later. And then there are women like Nancy and me.

I gained 70 pounds while pregnant with my twins. At three months along, my doctor said, "I'll give you a choice. Either work or work out—you can't do both." I chose work, because I knew I'd take time off with my new babies. While I still traveled around training clients, my own workouts were low-key: walking around the block, taking 10-minute swims, doing Kegels and pelvic tilts. Even so, after so many years of exercising, I thought for sure the weight would fall off me after my twins were born. But it took me a year and a half to get back my old shape.

Another thing that drove me crazy was hitting the plateaus. I'd be exercising, eating healthy foods, doing everything I know I'm supposed to do, and nothing happened. Then, two weeks later, I was suddenly down five or eight pounds. Then one pound came off, then maybe two, then another plateau. Those last 20 pounds were really tough to lose.

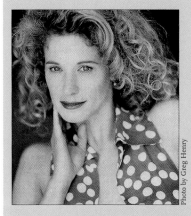

Nancy Travis

Allow your body some time to get back into shape. If you put yourself on an overly strict regimen, you're bound to go off it and then feel worse.

"I do as much activity as I can," Nancy says, "and at each stage, I try to build it up. The main thing is to do whatever little you can *consistently*." I agree.

Taking care of a little one means you have less time than ever for your workout, but you need it even more, especially the stress-reduction benefits. If you're creative, you can find ways to incorporate your offspring and his or her "equipment" into a decent workout.

To get back in shape while enjoying her new baby, Nancy bought a jogging stroller. She leashes up the dogs, puts on a backpack of baby essentials, and they all head out to a nearby park for a brisk two-mile walk and jog. "My baby loves it," she says. "He gets to look at all the people. And he can hear Mommy grunting behind him, so he knows I'm there."

You can make strolling with your baby into more of a workout by choosing a route with hills. Bring friends and hold a stroller aerobics class with side lunges, stretches, and other fun moves. (After all, you've done much sillier-looking things than this at aerobics class.)

When you're home and the baby's (finally!) asleep, you can add a quiet "hop and absorb" workout on the stairs, for both cardio and lower-body fitness. Another thing you can do is turn on an exercise video—yoga, step aerobics, abs—with the sound off. Just watch the screen and copy what they're doing. If you have an exercise bike or other quiet equipment at home, attach your baby monitor to it or near it. That way, you can hear if your child wakes up, but still focus on your workout.

THE INDISPENSABLE KEGEL EXERCISE

*One of the exercises that I teach all my female clients is the Kegel.
It's useful during pregnancy and after because it helps strengthen
the PC (pubococcygeal) muscle, which supports your uterus—
and which will be doing a lot of stretching for you during childbirth.*

*The PC muscle also supports your bladder and bowels, so it's not just
a muscle you worry about when you're pregnant. We've all seen those
ads for adult "shields" or diapers, and there's a reason for that.
Age, gravity, and babies weaken that muscle.*

*I've had clients worry about incontinence when they run or jump rope.
I remember one woman who took my aerobics classes, and always had to run
out and change afterwards because she'd wet her tights. Physical therapists
often recommend Kegels for women who experience such problems.*

Now that you're convinced, here's how to do the Kegel:

*Focus on the muscle you use to stop yourself from urinating—that's the
PC. (If you have trouble finding it, practice one or two squeezes in the
bathroom.) Squeeze that PC muscle, hold it for one second, then release.
Do 25 (or as many as you can to start). You can do this every day.*

*You can do Kegels in your car while commuting—at stoplights, for
example. Take a stick-on note, write "25 Kegels," and stick it in
your car by the speedometer. That will remind you to do them.*

This beats the usual routine of doing dishes and putting away toys, realizing you're exhausted and lying down—and then your child's nap is over. Instead, you'll have renewed energy. The dishes can wait.

I started working with Rob Lowe and his wife when they were expecting their first child, and I continued after the baby arrived.

At that point, Rob was preparing for a movie, *Frank and Jesse*, that demanded both acting talent and physical fitness—including riding horses and doing many of his own stunts. So he really needed to get in shape, but he wanted to spend as much time as possible with his wife, Cheryl, and their new baby.

As a lot of men do—you'd be surprised at how many!—Rob had put on some weight along with Cheryl during her pregnancy, so we focused on cardiovascular exercise. Rob wasn't used to doing 40 minutes of cardio. We'd alternate between the stationary bike and the treadmill, switching every 10 minutes to keep him motivated. Meanwhile, I worked with Cheryl on exercises to regain her prebaby shape and strength, focusing on abs, hips, thighs, and upper body.

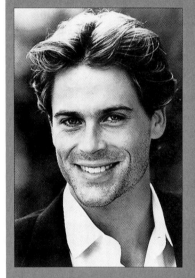

Rob Lowe

"We were in this little tiny gym—Cheryl, the baby, Kathy, me, and sometimes our dog, Sparky—and we still got a good workout," Rob recalls. "There were times when Cheryl was on the treadmill, and I'd be wrestling with the baby, or the other way around. Other times, we were both working out and Kathy was playing with the baby. That was like us training her for her future babies!"

When the dailies came back from *Frank and Jesse*, Rob was happy with how he looked, even in those shirtless scenes. But for him, working out is not just about looking good (he is naturally a very handsome man). "Whatever stress I'm feeling when I start my run or start playing full-court basketball, it's gone by the end," he says. "And that's what I need."

As a new parent, you have to be prepared for those times when everything falls apart. One day recently, the nanny who helps with my twins called in sick. I didn't want to cancel all my clients, so I improvised.

Instead of meeting my first client at the gym, she came to my house. I got my kids settled in bed in the guest room, put on a video for them, and she and I worked out in my little garage gym. There's a window from the guest room to the garage, so the boys could see me all the time (and vice versa). That was schedule-savior number one, because I could have easily just said, "Let's do it tomorrow."

My next client was a woman who has a six-month-old; turns out she didn't have child care either. She asked, "Could we go for a run? I'll put the baby in the jogger."

My two were now up and flying; on the way to meet her, I dropped off the twins at my mother-in-law's house, where she kindly watched them for an hour and a half.

You need to have that motivation to improve yourself. If exercise is truly a top priority, then you'll figure out ways to make it work. You might not have someone to watch your child all day, but there may be a relative or friend willing to take him for an hour. Find someone in the same boat, in one of those kids' classes, and trade—drop your kid with her in the morning for an hour, take a brisk walk, then take her child with you on errands later. That back-and-forth scheduling becomes another motivation to keep your exercise commitment.

> *"For me, getting pregnant was a go-ahead to eat whatever I wanted. It was the perfect excuse."*

Fitness While Traveling

When Michelle Pfeiffer wanted to keep fit on her family vacation, I told her to bring a jump rope. Jumping 10 minutes a day is a simple, total-body workout that's great for your heart and fun for your kids. And the rope is a cinch to pack. When I'm out of town, I aim for thirty minutes on a treadmill plus some sit-ups and push-ups in my room. That's enough to keep me from getting off track, so I won't feel I'm "starting over" when I get back home.

"Even just stretching on the floor of your hotel room is good," notes Nancy Travis. "When I'm doing TV shows, if I can't get to a gym, I run around the hotel. I don't feel embarrassed; I got over that."

"I find more people are getting into fitness; you won't be the only one running around. Mind you, you'll never see me in one of those little midriff tops with thong-style shorts!"

To expand your options, try to choose a hotel with or near a gym. When you're making reservations, ask what kind of facilities they have. Some have quite elaborate exercise rooms. For the same price, one hotel may have a gym while the other doesn't. Also, some hotels without gyms offer special discount rates to guests at a nearby health club. Make sure the gym has hours that work with your schedule.

If you'd like to do other exercises in your room, you could bring a list of the key movements on a sheet of paper to remind yourself. I'm always thinking of tricks that will call up a page from that mental encyclopedia of exercise that you can do wherever you are. In one of the first segments I did on *Today*, I demonstrated one memory tool. Using the word SILK, I created a lower-body workout with one exercise associated with each letter: Squat, Isolation (of pelvis), Lunge, and Kick-back. A lot of people called about that segment; they liked it and remembered it, so exercises came to them.

When you see something you'd like to do, whether it's on television, on a videotape, or at a class, it can be hard to recall the details. You're at the hotel or at your friend's house, wanting to keep fit, but your mind's a blank. Any little memory tricks you can come up with help. I remember, because this is what I do, but my clients don't remember unless I've worked with them as long as Michelle. And she'd better remember!

S.I.L.K.

Squat,
Isolation (of pelvis),
Lunge, and
Kick-back

Instructions

Squat
(for glutes and quads)
See page 96. Do 10.

Isolation
(for glutes, quads,
and lower abs)
Go down into a plié position:
Stand with your feet apart,
toes pointed outward, knees
bent over the toes, back
straight. Tilt your pelvis
forward 10 times.

Lunge
(for glutes, quads,
and hamstrings)
See page 64.
Do 10 on each leg.

Kick-back
(for quads
and hamstrings)
Stand facing the back of
a chair. Extend one leg back
slightly and kick your heel
toward your buttocks,
keeping your foot flexed.
Do 10 times on each leg.

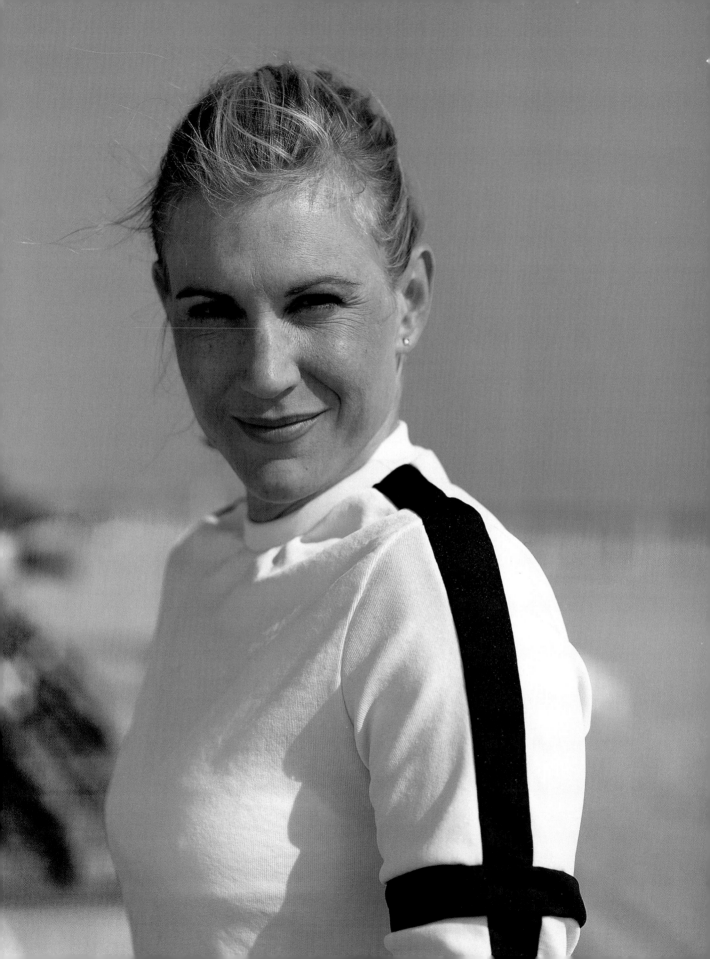

7 YOU'VE GOT IT— NOW KEEP IT!

STAYING MOTIVATED

A LOT OF MY CLIENTS START OUT WANTING LOOSER JEANS OR A SMALLER DRESS SIZE. OFTEN I SEE PEOPLE WHO TRY TO GET FIT AND SLIM TO PLEASE SOMEONE ELSE OR TO LOOK LIKE SOMEONE ELSE. BUT I PUSH THEM TO LOOK FOR MORE MEANINGFUL SIGNS OF IMPROVEMENT.

> I used to tell Kathy I'm too old to exercise, but now I find myself anxious for our next workout.
>
> —*Samuel L. Jackson*

I might point out to one client that when she started, she could do maybe 10 minutes on the Stairmaster—and now she can do 14. I constantly remind clients of those small improvements. I also take measurements, which are a much better way to see how a body's changing than looking at the scale. But most important, motivation has to be a personal thing. You won't work consistently to improve your body unless it's to please yourself.

When you see results, you're motivated to keep going. That's what happened to Michelle Pfeiffer. There are times for both Michelle and me when it's a drag to get up at 5:30. We may not be happy puppies when we get to the beach and start running. But eventually we'll realize we've gone four or five miles, and feel great.

Once Matt Lauer made time for regular workouts, he felt a night-and-day difference. "When I was not working out for a few years, I'd pick up a tennis racquet every once in a while. Three points later, I'd be gasping," he says. "And I'd be walking up the stairs to work and I'd be gasping. Now if I go skiing in the middle of the winter, even out West where the altitude is fairly high, I'm fine."

Al Roker gained new energy when he started regular workouts. "I just feel better at the end of the day. But there are days when you really have to push yourself to go. You know you'll feel better after. But while you're doing it . . . some days, I'm thinking my goal is just to be in great-enough shape that I can beat the crap out of my trainer and then never come back. Of course, that's just a fantasy . . ."

I recommended the same gym to both Matt Lauer and Al. "Getting there is not easy for me; it's thirty blocks from the *Today* studios, it's a car ride, and changing clothes, and then a car ride home," says Matt. "It's a bit of a pain in the neck, to be honest with you. But I find that even if I start to waver, and I start to think, Maybe I won't go today, because it's such a pain—if I can just drag myself there I'm always, always happier I did it when I'm walking out the door.

"I notice now that if I have a bad week or two weeks when I have to cancel out of workouts, I'm much worse for the wear and tear at the end of that time period," Matt says.

In a word, the secret to staying slim and fit is *consistency*. It's a lifestyle. Michelle Pfeiffer has been with me for seven years, Jami Gertz for eight, Julianne Phillips eight, and Penelope Ann Miller seven. It can be hard to stick with exercise, but it's much more difficult to stop altogether and start over again.

I love to be fit, to know what my body is capable of. As I'm writing this, I'm on vacation with my family in Canada. I had big plans: I would do 500 sit-ups and 100 push-ups a day. And I have yet to do one. We'll see if I get any done before I leave. I say every morning, "I'm gonna start doing my work." But it was 95 degrees today.

I'm in the same boat as other people: it's hard to start, but I love it by the time I'm done, and I love the results.

My sister-in-law was here last week. We both had our kids down for naps at the same time, so we walked six miles into town. I hadn't worked out for a week and a half before that. But I have strength and endurance because of the exercise I've been doing all my life. And that's what's important to me.

QUALITY OR QUANTITY?

Too much motivation and ambition can do more harm than good. "I've changed my fitness prescription over the years based upon research. In 1968 I said, More is better," Dr. Kenneth Cooper recalls. "But I stopped running marathons in 1969, because I listened to my body. It kept breaking down."

"By 1982 I was saying, If you run more than five miles a week, then you're running for something other than cardiovascular fitness. Beyond that point, you don't get as much improvement in your aerobic capacity. And the number of musculoskeletal injuries increase dramatically."

Julianne Phillips, who thrives on physical challenge, used to feel guilty if she didn't work out seven days a week. Now

On Sunday, I put on water skis, got behind my uncle's boat, and was able to slalom for five minutes. I'm paying for it today; my whole upper body is sore. But I know I can step onto skis when I haven't done it for 364 days, and I can do it. I love that feeling.

For some people, looking forward to that good feeling from exercise isn't enough. For them, a focus on the health consequences of being inactive may help. "Some people can find more fun ways to do it, but some people will never like exercise," says Dr. Andrea Dunn. "None of us likes flossing our teeth either, but quite a few of us do it because we don't want to suffer the consequences of having our gums scraped."

"On weekends, I play tennis with guys twenty or thirty years older than me," Rob Lowe told me recently. "I'm impressed with how they keep themselves together, and I want to be like that. And there's only one way to get it."

REWARD YOURSELF

One of the exercise-motivating tricks Dr. Andrea Dunn recommends is finding which rewards work for you. "We try to get people to think of the intangibles as well as the tangible things," she says. "We had a client who said, 'If I meet my physical activity goals for the year, well, I've wanted to take a walking vacation in Ireland.' Every week she did it, she'd put money in the piggy bank for her trip. And pretty soon, she'd done it. She had enough money to go, and she was fit enough to go."

Another woman's reward strategy involved an agreement with her husband that he'd pay her for doing her walking. Eventually, she was walking so much that they had to renegotiate.

"A third woman got her friends at church together and they formed a walking group," Dr. Dunn adds. "If people didn't walk, they had to put money in the pot. Every three months, whoever had shown up the most got the money that was in the pot."

Says Claudia Schiffer, "Music always keeps me motivated, as much as the good feeling I get after exercise. I think it also has a lot to do with stress relief." Claudia treated herself to a nice belt for her Walkman so she wouldn't have to carry it in her hand.

What inspires Rita Wilson the most is just knowing how many calories she's burning per workout. "I know how hard I have to exercise to burn 500 calories," she explains. "I also know how easy it is to eat 500 calories, and that helps me not to cheat during the day."

she aims for five or six. "Life is too short; there are too many things to do. And I've learned that it's about quality, not necessarily quantity. On the days that I feel like I *have* to work out, I don't do it."

Julianne also has those days when she wakes up tired, and doesn't feel motivated. "You have to be able to distinguish between procrastination and your body needing a break."

The American College of Sports Medicine recommends fairly vigorous exercise for 20 to 60 minutes a day, three to five days a week. But it also promotes rest as a crucial part of that routine (assuming you've done something to rest up from!). For exercises that stress the muscles, the college encourages a day of rest after every two or three days of training.

Falling into Old Habits— and Getting Back on Track

Preventing exercise "relapse" is another thing that Andrea Dunn talks about with her clients at the Cooper Institute. "Take the stereotypical example of the person who joins a gym at New Year's. She goes faithfully for the first three weeks. Then she misses a session in the fourth week, but she still goes back.

"Then she misses two sessions in the sixth week," Dr. Dunn continues. "And pretty soon, by the end of the second month, she's decided, 'Well, I've missed some sessions, and I'm destined to fail—so I might just as well not do it.' We try to get people to stop thinking like that."

Penelope Ann Miller finds that being consistent helps. "If I go off for a few days I notice that it's much harder to start back into a routine," she says. "Once I'm on a roll, I'm really good about staying with it, but if I stop for a few days and procrastinate or something comes up, it's definitely harder to get going again. I sort of have to force myself. And once I get going, I love it, and then I'm back into a groove."

Dr. Dunn points out that some cycling in and out of activity is common. "The thing is to be persistent in your efforts and keep trying," she says. "And pretty soon, you're going to find what works for you."

"The best time for me to exercise is right after *Today*, because the longer I put off working out, the better the chances are I'll find some wonderful excuse not to go," says Al Roker. "It's I've got this meeting, I've gotta go to a lunch, I've got to get ready for the five o'clock news ...' And that way, of course, you get more and more out of shape. And the more you get out of shape, the worse you feel."

When you're trying to change ingrained daily habits, such as patterns of activity and exercise, it takes effort, and failure, and renewed effort. "Most people who quit smoking haven't done it in one attempt," Dr. Dunn points out.

One trick is to plan ahead for times when you might relapse. The schedule disruptions that come with business travel or family visits, for example. Think of specific things you can do to maintain your exercise habits during those times.

Keep It Interesting

FITNESS WITH A PARTNER OR GROUP

The secret to Jami Gertz's exercise routine is a sense of humor. "If you can't laugh at yourself, it's hard to imagine getting anywhere," she points out. For Jami, having a workout partner to laugh with keeps her motivated and entertained.

I do the same thing with Billy. When we go to the park with our kids, he'll run over to the pull-up bar and say, "Let's see how many you've got today!" He always feels he has to do one more than me, and I threaten to make him go first.

"For me, the most important thing was finding somebody to work out with who was flexible, and whom I liked spending time with," says Matt Lauer. "I would tire very quickly of spending an hour working out with someone I didn't want to talk to." This is true whether you use a trainer, as Matt does, or exercise with a friend, spouse, or group.

"What I find hard to do is just getting up and going somewhere," says Penelope Ann Miller, "so that's why I like having Kathy come to me. Or I schedule time to play tennis with friends, or take a hike with friends and our dogs. That makes it fun, and I'm not thinking, This hour I have to go to a gym and get dressed and all that. This way I'm more consistent with exercise."

Andrea Dunn teaches her clients at the Cooper Institute how to scout for opportunities to get active in their communities, especially ones that will also provide social support. "One of the people in our current research study found out about a walking group called the Dallas Trekkers," she says. "She started going on the walks. She liked the people so much that now she's running for president of one of the chapters. She's got her whole fitness support system built in."

"There are people who really need that group support, and like it. If that's what they need and like, that's what they should do," Dr. Dunn adds. "There are others—I'm one of them—who don't really enjoy working out with groups of people. I like to keep that as my time to think."

If you do have a spouse or good friend to work out with, use each other as exercise equipment. Try resistance exercises on each other. Do modified push-ups (you push

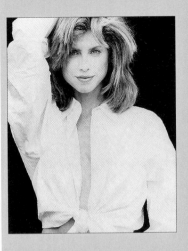

On those days I don't want to go work out, Kathy flashes through my mind. She has the twins, flies back and forth to New York all the time, and she never seems tired. And I tell myself, "C'mon, get your big butt off this chair and get workin'!"

—*Julianne Phillips*

while your partner applies light pressure to your back). You can also do partner stretching. I did this one with Samuel L. Jackson after our first workout together: Stand behind your partner, facing his back. Have him extend his arms out to the side. Then, attach your hands to his, and stretch his arms backward, until he feels it through the front of his chest and shoulders.

Social support can make things easier as you're trying to create the fitness habit. It's not essential to have someone to walk with you, but most people do better with someone they can talk to about their goals and progress. They can remind you to do it, or reinforce you for doing it with some good words: "I'm proud of you. I'm impressed!" Having someone to cheer you on can make the difference.

VARYING YOUR ROUTINE

To keep Rita Wilson from getting bored as she toned up for her role in the movie *Jingle All the Way*, I varied her routine. One day we'd do an hour of hiking, followed by abdominal work. On others, there were step aerobics, lunges in the sand, running, fast walking, or body-sculpting with weights. Rita was ecstatic with the results.

Candice Bergen would always tell me that she liked to have exercises over with very quickly. She didn't want to reduce our training time, just the time spent on the individual exercises. Going outside to walk was one thing, but walking in place for 30 minutes on the treadmill got dull, even if we varied the speed to make it challenging. It made the workout seem much longer for her.

So we developed our own kind of circuit training. If she walked on the treadmill, I'd take her off after five minutes to do something else. Time went by really quickly that way.

Breaking up a workout is now something I do with other clients. We'll do the five minutes on the treadmill or bike, then spend five on jumping rope, doing lunges across the floor, or upper-body work with pliés: a variety of moves to keep the heart rate up and work different muscle groups. Then, it's back on the bike for five. This keeps my clients stimulated mentally and physically, and cuts down on clock-watching.

"I also like breaking it up," says Penelope Ann Miller. "I don't like the same kind of workout. I love to swim, and walk, and hike, play tennis, and bike-ride. I just bought a mountain bike. I'm trying, especially this summer, to do something every day that's really fun."

"With Kathy, sometimes I'll do the treadmill or the step aerobics or the Stairmaster," she says. "We'll do the jump rope, and then leg exercises, then stomach exercises or something with the ball or the bands. She's always mixing it up."

"I'M BORED": UNCOMMON EXERCISES

When a friend suggested that I might enjoy a Tae Bo class, my first thoughts were, What the heck is Tae Bo? and There's no way I'm driving from Beverly Hills to the San Fernando Valley to get some exercise! Tae Bo, it turned out, is a combination of Tae Kwan Do, aerobics, and kick boxing. Adding this variation to my usual workouts not only helped me lose that last 20 pounds from my pregnancy, it revitalized my interest and kicked me into higher gear.

When Michelle Pfeiffer trained for the very physical role of Catwoman, kick boxing was part of her routine. "It really is a lot of fun," she says, "and a really good workout. I had to continue with it because of the movie, but I wouldn't rely on it for a regular workout. My body was getting too battered—I was injuring and reinjuring my hamstrings. You just have to be careful with it."

Regular boxing is another variation. It's a lot like the kind of training session a professional boxer would go through: you learn how to spar, hit the punching bag, jump rope, and do rounds of calisthenics such as push-ups and sit-ups. It's fun, it's different, and for me, it's a great stress reliever. I enjoy the challenge of developing skills, from self-defense moves to just the right way to execute a hit.

Developing a skill takes your brain away from "How many calories am I burning? How much longer do I have?" It's not like treading on the Stairmaster, watching the minutes and seconds tick down. While the Stairmaster gives a good workout, it's not exactly mentally challenging.

Another sport involving lots of skill is fencing. I did a fencing segment on *Today*. An instructor from New York's Chelsea Piers put me through a lesson, then came on the show with me to talk about fencing as exercise. As we demonstrated basic technique,

EXERCISE LIKE A KID

Most of us loved running and jumping as children. Thinking back to your favorite childhood games can be a secret fitness weapon, helping you find an exercise plan you can stick with. Did you like jumping rope or helping out in the garden? Did you swim almost every summer day?

One example is snow or sand angels. Remember rushing out into the snow, falling back, and making a snow angel? You didn't worry about your thighs back then, but today the same motion can help you get fit. Lie in the snow or sand, with arms at your side and legs together. In a continuous motion, push the sand away from you, then pull it back to your starting position. Do 20 of these.

I could feel the muscles in my legs working; the stance (knees bent, back straight) calls on lower body strength.

Another benefit: the equipment looks really cool. And if your kids are fans of Zorro or *Star Wars* (they fenced with those lightsabers), they'll be so impressed.

Learn to Love (or at Least Get Along with) Your Body

La Tanya Richardson told me she wanted to look like Michelle Pfeiffer. She said, "I'm paying you, so you should make me look like this!" But I just laughed, as if to say, "I know you're not serious, and I'm not serious. But you know the answer." LaTanya and I have an understanding now that where we're coming from is, How can she feel really good? How can she be the best that she can be?

People do hire me and say, "If I do that, will I look like Michelle? Will I look like you?" It would be nice to say, "Perhaps, if you do these exercises as often as you can, get in enough cardio work, and eat well." But that's lame. I say straight out, "Your legs won't look like mine. These are my legs, those are yours. But you clearly can improve what you have, just as I have."

That's why I hate doing magazine interviews where they'll ask, "Give us the secret to Jennifer Aniston's flat stomach!" It encourages people to emulate someone they're not. I can understand the curiosity about what stars do, but the real question is, How can you make what you have the best it can be?

A big problem with women is that we rarely look at what we *do* enjoy about our bodies. If you're putting yourself down 99 percent of the time, how are you ever going to think positively about what you're doing?

I am constantly asked, "Is this exercise gonna give me a smaller rear?" or slimmer hips, or whatever they imagine is their worst feature. While a lot can be accomplished with exercise, a change in your point of view is also powerful medicine.

When LaTanya moved with her husband, Samuel L. Jackson, from New York to Los Angeles, she felt increasingly self-conscious. "Walking around New York, you have a greater sense of your body in motion. In California, there's a greater focus on what it looks like. I'd never been that conscious of my looks, but when you see what is accepted, and you know you don't fit that . . . I was beating myself up with this."

"Kathy helped me see it was bad thinking," LaTanya adds. "That's not what your body is for. Those are emaciated frames people have starved themselves into, not working machines. You don't need a body like that to be healthy and happy, and to perform."

It's hard to overcome those years of media conditioning on what bodies should be— especially for women, though men are starting to feel that pressure, too. I know LaTanya will sometimes compare her looks to a picture she has of herself, which is certainly more positive than wanting to look like someone else.

"It's hard because I'm older; I keep thinking about how I looked when I was young," says LaTanya, "but I probably didn't even look like that."

"If I do that, will I look like Michelle? Will I look like you?"

There's a "look" out there in the media that women feel they need to live up to. But it's a fantasy, even for those polished cover-girl beauties; they get that look through computer imaging, makeup, and the rest of the tricks. We think we're supposed to look like something that's not real. In my first years of college, even I was caught up in this trap; I'd pin up photos of actresses or models in my dorm room as a guide to what I wanted to look like.

Realize that in this century, "ideal" body measurements have veered all over the place: wide hips and tiny waist, skinny and flat all over, sculpted muscles with big breasts . . . you get the picture. Sometimes (like today) the ideal is so out of whack with women's real bodies that most of us would need plastic surgery to achieve it. (In the "hourglass" figure era, a few women actually had their lower ribs removed so they could pull that corset tighter.)

"I don't know anyone who thinks they have a perfect body," says Nancy Travis. "People in this business have to know that they're being photographed in the most flattering ways, and dressed specially, with teams of people to help them look great."

For example, I was recently on the cover of a magazine, and you would hardly know it was me. They had to touch up my arms: they're muscular but looked flat and fat in the photo.

"I look at models and think, 'Gosh, I wonder how many sit-ups it would take?' But I actually have come to a place where I really like my body. Instead of it being an external thing, it's more how I feel inside: healthy and confident," says Nancy. "It comes from balancing all the areas in my life, without being too strict in any one. I let myself be."

Even supermodels need to do that. "I learned that exercise is not only about creating a muscular body," Claudia Schiffer says. "It's also about your mind, your confidence, and your self-esteem."

Eating Well

Diet fads come and go: the Zone, the blood-type diet, the Scarsdale diet, the cabbage-soup diet. "People follow what's popular in the magazines and books," says Michelle Daum, a registered dietitian and former chief clinical nutritionist at the North Shore University–Cornell University Medical College in New York. "A very intelligent woman I know said to me, to my surprise, that the cabbage-soup diet works. By that she meant that it does what it says it's going to do: she lost pounds quickly. The fact that it was mostly just water loss, and that she immediately regained the weight, was irrelevant to her." It doesn't last, and often you gain back what you lost—plus!

Dr. Daniel Kosich, exercise science editor for *Shape* magazine, blames many failed attempts on overly rigid food plans: "Here's what I'll eat this week for breakfast, lunch, and dinner." Those don't last long. Strict eating rules are likely to backfire, leaving you more obsessed with food than ever. Food shouldn't be a love-hate relationship—like those magazine covers piled with gooey desserts, promoting the latest diet.

"It's more realistic to recognize that there aren't really good and bad foods," says Dr. Kosich. "Some foods are packed with nutrients and some are dense with calories. The challenge is to have most of your diet come from fruits, veggies, and whole grains, and a small amount from those foods most people know not to use in excess."

YOU'RE NOT ALONE

Michelle Daum told me about a client of hers who felt, as many heavy people do, that thinness comes naturally to everyone else: they can eat whatever they want and not gain a pound, while she has to deprive herself.

Michelle suggests, "Next time you go out to eat, look carefully at what the other, thinner women are ordering for lunch. Most will be having salads. And that thin woman over there, enjoying the gooey dessert—she doesn't eat that way all day, every day. She may have had a very light lunch or gone for a jog that afternoon to allow herself that cheesecake."

It's not just the chubby who need to eat with balance and moderation—it's pretty much everybody.

DON'T SABOTAGE YOUR WORKOUTS

"I remember the stupid stuff I did growing up,"
says LaTanya Richardson. "We used to just
not eat. We had unhealthy habits, smoked
cigarettes—I was fine with a cigarette and a cup
of coffee. Later, my focus became more on
a healthy, strong, leaner body."

"I was a really heavy smoker for
a long time," admits Michelle Pfeiffer.
"And when I quit, I plunged into exercise."

Michelle never smoked around me,
and she hasn't smoked now for years.
But I have had clients who smoke.
Some of my current clients will
smoke when they go out to parties.

My feeling about smoking is,
Why bother? That's really how I feel.
Why bother to exercise when you're
going to smoke? I know people who
do run and smoke, probably thinking,
Well, if I work out, that will lessen my risk.
But to me, I just can't imagine doing both.

If you smoke, my hope is that exercise
might help you realize how bad smoking
is for you. You may feel its effects in
your lungs, get a wake-up call, and
realize it just doesn't work.

"Most evidence supports the food pyramid approach: mostly carbohydrates, 20 to 30 percent fat, 15 to 20 percent protein," he adds. "In the short term there's little health risk from a high-protein (over 20 percent) diet. But in the long run, it's associated with kidney problems and osteoporosis."

Saturated fat should be no more than 10 percent of your day's calories. Try using more olive oil and less butter or margarine in your cooking.

"I DON'T LIKE BREAKFAST"

Sometimes simple things, such as changing the times of day that you eat or eating slowly, can make a surprising difference. Dr. Kosich recommends eating 65 to 70 percent of your calories before your last meal of the day.

"Kathy gets mad because I don't like breakfast or lunch! I'm only hungry at dinner," says Penelope Ann Miller. "And she says, 'It's not good for you; your body needs the fuel, and it starts working once you feed it.' So I try to have three balanced meals, and just not overdo it. I'll have a protein shake in the morning and force myself to have lunch—a tuna sandwich or something. Then I'm not as hungry at dinner."

"About one-third of my clients don't want breakfast; they have coffee and they're fine," says Michelle Daum. "I insist, though, that they eat by lunchtime. They worry that eating in the morning will set them off to overeat all day. But if you eat no breakfast and lunch, by 4:00 P.M. you'll eat everything in the fridge."

"One of the worst habits of overweight individuals is they skip breakfast, skip lunch, start eating at 4:00 or 5:00 P.M.—and eat continually and excessively until bedtime," adds Michelle. "Then, they're not hungry in the morning. It's the worst eating pattern possible." If you're not sure you'll have healthy food around during the day, bring some.

TAKE IT SLOWLY

What, when, and why you eat are deeply engrained habits. Suppose you decide, From now on, I'll eat three healthy meals a day and have only fruit for snacks! But if you've been eating Egg McWhatsits for breakfast and fast-food burgers and fries for lunch

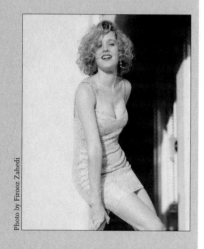

Photo by Firooz Zahedi

I never diet. Because the minute your mind thinks you're dieting, you feel deprived and then you're starving and you crave things. I just try to eat right, in moderation. I'm not the kind of person who says, "I'll never eat sugar or never eat fat." I just don't think you can do that.

—*Penelope Ann Miller*

and dinner, no matter how seriously you vow, it's not likely to stick. It's too big and too sudden a change. You'll end up feeling like a failure and go eat a pint of ice cream.

Instead of setting yourself up for a fall, take it in manageable steps. In the first few weeks, have fast food for lunch and dinner, but make a good breakfast at home of oatmeal and fruit. After a few weeks, have the burger at lunch, but make a grilled chicken breast and fresh vegetables at home for dinner. It's a silly example, I know, but this is how you change eating habits for life: start small, go slowly, be realistic. Buy the smaller-size chocolate bar; have fresh fruit for dessert one night a week.

When I got out of college, I felt as if I were addicted to Diet Coke. The 7-Eleven was just down the block, and we'd get Big Gulps; just one is like a six-pack of cans. I knew I had to wean myself off this.

I allowed myself one Big Gulp a day; when I couldn't wait any longer, I'd go get it. The rest of the time, I drank sparkling water. Slowly, the Big Gulp gave way to the Large, the Large became the Medium, I was drinking more bottled water ... and eventually, I didn't have that strong craving anymore.

PORTIONS

Eating well doesn't have to be complicated. I just eat in moderation. Not a lot of sweets, but lots of vegetables, fruits, chicken, and pasta. I have oatmeal for breakfast. One problem is that most of us have never learned about portion size. We finish all the food on our plates, even when we're too full. Get in the habit of leaving food on your plate.

"If I'm working with sometime who has to eat out consistently, like cops on the beat who buy lunch out every day, I tell them, 'Take what you're currently eating and cut it down by one-third, or one-fourth," says Michelle Daum. "It's not ideal, but even if you get a bacon cheeseburger and fries, if you leave one-third uneaten, it will do the job."

LaTanya Richardson hates to see food go to waste. She has a teenager who has friends over, which means lots of food around. Also, because she and her husband are in the entertainment business, gifts (including food) are frequently sent to their house. She has a very hard time just taking whatever's left over and throwing it out or giving it away.

"Forget what your mother told you," says Michelle. "The kids in India won't get that food, and your heart will suffer if you do. It's your health or the trash can."

You don't need to buy a calorie counter or a food scale: just estimate. For example, a serving of chicken or fish should be no bigger than the palm of your hand. A pasta portion should fit into your cupped hands.

Portion control is also an issue for LaTanya. "To take weight off, I have to eat five meals a day, little portions, vegetables and fruit mostly," she says. "Like this morning I had oatmeal and grapefruit. I'll make as many greens as I can fit on a plate, with peppers plus a little olive oil and balsamic vinegar, and it's delicious. If you don't eat often, you get too hungry."

COPING WITH CRAVINGS

"Sometimes I'll say to Kathy, 'God, I'm craving a burger,'" confides Alfre Woodard. "And she says, 'Then just have half a burger, and you'll forget about it.' She's very practical."

I'm not big on cookies or cake, but I like chocolate, and I like 1950s-style American food: mashed potatoes, grilled cheese sandwiches, waffles with butter and syrup, all that good food. And I hate to feel deprived. I don't want to know I can't have a grilled cheese sandwich. So I don't have the attitude that I'll never have them; I just have them less often. And when I do, I have a small portion and am satisfied with that.

If you see something that you feel you've got to have, like chocolate, try to get into this mind-set: "There's always going to be chocolate—and there'll be better chocolate. I'm not gonna die if I don't eat that. That's not the last piece in the world." Then you can just take a bite and leave the rest. It helps me to pass something by if I can have a small portion or a bite. When my kids go to McDonald's, I grab a couple of their fries.

"I'm from Texas, so if you offered me a plate of chocolate chip cookies or a plate of hamburger patties, I'd want the hamburger," says Peri Gilpin. "So I really look forward to a lean meal with protein in meat form."

Peri just eats more chicken and fish for dinner, and less beef. "There are so many things that you love that you can have in a day. Well, you can't have a piece of cheesecake every day—but you can have it once a week."

Don't try to give up snacks and treats altogether. Fresh fruit or vegetables are great, of course. But now and then have some of what you really want. "I have one patient who lost about 45 pounds. Every afternoon around four o'clock, she would have a snack-size Milky Way bar. It took the edge off, and she was happy," says Michelle Daum. "But some people will say, 'I can't have just one, it will get me started.' Know your weaknesses."

Portion control helps make cravings manageable. Another client of Michelle's was able to stop munching on the holiday candy she bought for her kids by putting it in little bags with ribbon ties. You might also get freezable snacks—take out one a day to thaw, and leave the rest in the freezer.

But when you give in too much to a craving, don't beat yourself up. Don't dwell on it. It's okay. That's life. Everyone has bad days. It's easy to get right back on track if you don't obsess about it and dig a deeper hole.

As Dr. Daniel Kosich says, don't look at just that day's calories. Focus on your energy intake and output over time, perhaps week by week. "To lose a pound this week, you must expend 3500 calories," he notes. "It doesn't matter to your body exactly how you do it."

WORKING GOOD EATING HABITS INTO YOUR LIFE

Here are other tips from Michelle Daum, and from me:

- Cut out the caloric beverages

  This includes the Snapples, Arizona Iced Teas, soft drinks, and lemonades. Watch out for the ones that look clear and calorie-free, but aren't (check the label). Also beware those new calorie-packed coffee drinks. (If you crave one, ask for it with nonfat milk.)

  Plain spring water is great, but it can get boring. No-calorie sparkling water with flavor essence added is okay, or squeeze in some lemon or lime. You can also feel like you're getting a treat by adding an ounce of diet soda or Crystal Lite to your fizzy water.

I'll take out a large bottle of seltzer, and splash in a little ginger ale (regular or diet)—about a 10-to-one ratio of seltzer to ginger ale. But my rule is that I have to drink all of that water. I do the same for my twins, adding a splash of apple juice to their water. You can also freeze fruit juice into ice cubes, and use the cubes to pep up your H_2O.

- Have healthy snacks ready and waiting

When you come home starving at the end of a long day, it's too easy to rip open the cookies or chips. Michelle Daum recommends, "Have some gazpacho ready in the fridge. You can buy it, or make it yourself; just cut up some veggies in tomato juice."

Gazpacho is crunchy and refreshing. You can make a big Tupperware bowl of it and use it all week. When I was doing spa research for Jane Fonda at the Golden Door, they served gazpacho as a midday snack, and it was great.

You just want something that will take the edge off your hunger, so you're less likely to munch before dinner. Cut-up vegetables are also good, along with "fast food" fruit like grapes or bananas.

- Don't eat from your kids' plates

New moms especially have difficulty with this. I was right up there with them, nibbling on the mac-and-cheese, grilled cheese sandwiches, and those other toddler favorites. It's so easy to say, 'You take a bite and Mom will take a bite.' Then, I'd go have dinner, and never even think about the extra I'd been eating.

- Sit down

Michelle Daum recommended this trick to a gourmet cook who weighed 250 pounds and nibbled constantly while preparing dinner. "At 4:00, I'd have her sit down at a table with a cup of tea and an elegant snack on a pretty little plate, with garnish." That special snack satisfied her mentally and physically.

When I can find (or make) time for a sit-down lunch, those are always the days that I do really well. I don't consider snacking, I have energy, and feel clear and focused: just from sitting down for 30 minutes. It's like a message to your brain: I am sitting. I am eating. Now I am full. When you walk past the table and stuff something in your mouth, or run by the store and grab a snack, you're not aware of how much you're eating.

- Be a "reduced-fat" skeptic

"I didn't get too much into that whole nonfat thing, where everything's packed with sugar—thank goodness," says Peri Gilpin.

The "reduced-fat" label is so enticing, but it tempts you to eat more than you'd dare otherwise, wiping out any benefits.

Often, the calorie difference between regular and reduced-fat is trivial.

"A regular Oreo has 53 calories; a reduced-fat one has 50," notes Michelle Daum. "I personally hate nonfat cream cheese and all that other fake stuff. I'd rather use real olive oil, only a little, than use diet dressing."

I agree—use the real stuff, not the reduced-fat, but in moderation. One exception is low-fat dairy products, which *are* the real thing. If you don't like nonfat milk, go with one-percent. It's a great source of nutrients, especially calcium for your bones.

- Eat a healthier lunch

If you eat out a lot, try to brown-bag it twice a week. You have more control over what you eat. Pack a sandwich, fruit, and little snack: a small cookie or two (such as Chips Ahoy), pretzels, or a snack-size candy bar. Alternatives include cut-up vegetables, low-fat or nonfat yogurt (not too sugary), a bag of low-oil popcorn, or unsweetened rice cakes. Go easy on the processed foods, like Lunchables.

If you have to eat out, a salad with grilled chicken (dressing on the side) is usually good. Even at a diner, you can get a turkey sandwich or roast chicken and a baked potato (one pat of butter, or a small dab of sour cream).

Another great tip for eating out is to share an entree. Our country is just out of whack with portion sizes; American restaurants are the worst. A correct portion size looks paltry in comparison, but it's what your body is normally capable of eating. Sharing gives you the right amount. It's especially good with higher-fat foods; share the burger and have salad on the side. If you really want one, split a dessert (it's the first few bites that taste best, anyway).

- Navigate travel eating

Plan ahead. You wouldn't take a child on a three-hour car or plane trip with no food, so do the same for yourself. Get an insulated lunch sack with a little cold pack, and bring a turkey sandwich with mustard and tomato, plus some fresh fruit. When you take that out on the plane, you'll get envious looks. This also works for sports events (no more expensive, greasy hot dogs).

When you're on a family vacation, avoid those buffets. I know in Las Vegas, it's everywhere you turn: "$2.99 — All You Can Eat!" inviting you to stuff yourself with grease and starch. All that food is overwhelming, and your brain forgets to signal that you're full.

Are You Ready to Change?

One thing that Dr. Andrea Dunn has learned about fitness is that "people change at different rates. And one thing that works for one person isn't going to work for everybody else."

To help get her clients at the Cooper Institute clear on their motivations to change, she leads them through a series of steps. I've done my own version of them here. If you think it would help you set goals and keep motivated, write down your responses.

- What are some *specific risks* (disease, disability, self-dislike, social consequences, and so on) that you feel you personally could avoid through regular exercise?

- What are some *specific benefits* (improved health, reduced stress, happier social life, and so on) that you believe you could gain through regular exercise? (Review "Why do you want to get fit?" in Chapter 1.)

- What are some ways your *family and friends* might benefit if you're more physically active? For example, playing outside or walking with your children creates good memories and passes on the fitness habit. Walks with your spouse give you quiet time for talking.

"People change at different rates. And one thing that works for one person isn't going to work for everybody else."

- What kinds of *opportunities* could you realistically take advantage of to add activity to your week? Think about each part of your day, emphasizing those times when you're often stressed or tired. (Review the ideas in Chapter 2, "Stealth Fitness.")

- *Who can you find to help you* get more exercise? This might be a spouse, friend, or co-worker. Don't forget that neighborhood parent who could trade child care with you.

- What ways can you *reward yourself* for meeting goals? Do you want to put money away every week for a walking or skiing vacation? Will fitting into your old jeans make you wanna dance?

- How can you set up *reminders* to carry out your goals? You might try sticky notes, computer-clock alarms, or appointments with walking partners.

Consider taking time each week to make an activity plan. Write down when and where you plan to add physical movement to your days, and the kinds you plan to do.

I'm encouraged when I think about how far we've come even to have exercise as a topic people talk about. We've had Jane Fonda with aerobic dancing to music, "going for the burn," Richard Simmons, Kathy Smith, Denise Austin—many pioneers entering the marketplace with wonderful programs that have gradually created an awareness of the benefits of fitness.

But there are still alarming numbers of Americans who are not active. I'd love to be known as someone who helped to change that. That's what it's really about. Getting the family outdoors after dinner, parking a few blocks away from the store, skipping that moving walkway at the airport—there are so many places each day to discover healthy activity. If this book does nothing but lead you to take the stairs instead of the elevator on a regular basis, I'll consider it a success.

These simple changes offer incredible benefits to your health, your work, your independence, and the people you care for.

APPENDIX

Where Can I Find Out More About ...

There's always more to learn, especially if you want to keep motivated and fresh.
Here are some of my favorite sources for fitness and health information and support.

BOOKS

The Aerobics Program for Total Well-being: Exercise, Diet and Emotional Balance, by Kenneth Cooper, M.D. (Bantam Doubleday Dell, 1985). A comprehensive book by one of the pioneers of aerobic fitness.

The Can-Do Eating Plan for Overweight Kids and Teens, by Michelle Daum, M.S., R.D., with Amy Lemley. (Avon Books, 1997). Useful ideas, and not just for kids.

Primetime Pregnancy, by Kathy Kaehler and Cynthia Tivers (Contemporary Books, 1998). More exercises and ideas for a healthy, safe pregnancy (plus more photos of how huge I looked pregnant with twins).

Get Real: A Personal Guide to Real-Life Weight Management, by Daniel Kosich, Ph.D. (International Association of Fitness Professionals, San Diego, 1995).

VIDEOS

The Kathy Kaehler Fitness System (Columbia Tristar)

Versa Training Abs and Legs (Reebok)

Target and Tone (CBS/Fox)

The Perfectly Fit Series (four videos on different body areas) with Claudia Schiffer (CBS/Fox)

INTERNET SITES

• You can e-mail me at kathykaehler@earthlink.net

• *Today*: www.msnbc.com. Click on "On Air."

• The Centers for Disease Control and Prevention, National Center for Chronic Disease Prevention and Health Promotion, Division of Nutrition and Physical Activity: www.cdc.gov. The whole CDC site has all kinds of useful information for the public about health topics.

A summary of results from *Physical Activity and Health: A Report of the Surgeon General* and an order form for the whole report are available online at www.cdc.gov/nccdphp/sgr/sgr.htm. (This is written for the public as well as for academics.) You can also get information from the CDC (toll-free) by calling 1-888-232-4674.

• *The Journal of the American Medical Association*'s Web site (www.ama-assn.org/public/journals/jama/jamahome.htm) has health information for the public, searchable by topic, in Science News Update (click on "latest news") and the Patient Page.

ACADEMIC JOURNALS

Here are a few of the research articles we relied on in this book. You can usually find them at the nearest medical or college library. You may also look up these and other references through MEDLINE, a free medical information search service of the National Institutes of Health, at www.ncbi.nlm.nih.gov/PubMed.

• Steven Blair, James Kampert, Harold Kohl III, et al., "Influences of cardiorespiratory fitness and other precursors on cardiovasular disease and all-cause mortality in men and women." *Journal of the American Medical Association*, July 17, 1996, pages 205–210.

• Steven Blair, "Evidence for success of exercise in weight loss and control." *Annals of Internal Medicine*, October 1, 1993, pages 702–706.

• Steven Blair, Harold Kohl III, Ralph Paffenbarger Jr., et al., "Physical fitness and all-cause mortality." *Journal of the American Medical Association*, November 3, 1989, pages 2395–2401.

• Kelly Brownell, Albert Stunkard, and Janet Michelle Albaum, "Evaluation and modification of exercise patterns in the natural environment." *American Journal of Psychiatry*, December 1980, pages 1540–1545.

• John Duncan, Neil Gordon, and Chris Scott, "Women walking for health and fitness: how much is enough?" *Journal of the American Medical Association*, December 18, 1991, pages 3295–3299.

• Andrea Dunn, Melissa Garcia, Bess Marcus, et al., "Six-month physical activity and fitness changes in Project Active, a randomized trial." *Medicine & Science in Sports & Exercise*, July 1998, pages 1076–1083.

• Andrea Dunn, Bess Marcus, James Kampert, et al., "Reduction in cardiovascular disease risk factors: 6-month results from Project Active." *Preventive Medicine*, November 1997, pages 883–892.

• Andrea Dunn, "Getting started—a review of physical activity adoption studies." *British Journal of Sports Medicine*, September 1996, pages 193–199.

• M. H. Murphy and A. E. Hardman, "Training effects of short and long bouts of brisk walking in sedentary women." *Medicine & Science in Sports & Exercise*, January 1998, pages 152–157.

• Anthony Vita, Richard Terry, Helen Hubert, and James Fries, "Aging, health risks, and cumulative disability." *The New England Journal of Medicine*, April 9, 1998, pages 1035–1041.

Notes